From Medicine to Psychotherapy

Mark O. Aveline, MD, FRCPsych, DPM

Consultant Psychotherapist, Nottingham Health Authority
Clinical Teacher, University of Nottingham

Psychotherapy Series

Series editor: **Windy Dryden**

Foreword by R.F. Hobson, BA, MD, FRCPsych, DPM

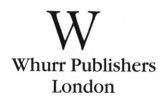

Whurr Publishers
London

First published 1992 by
Whurr Publishers Ltd
19b Compton Terrace, London N1 2UN, England

British Library Cataloguing in Publication Data
Aveline, Mark
  From medicine to psychotherapy.
  I. Title
  616.89

  ISBN 1-870332-58-X

Typeset by Inforum Typesetting, Portsmouth
Printed and bound in the UK by Athenaeum Press Ltd, Newcastle upon Tyne

From Medicine
to Psychotherapy

The Whurr Psychotherapy Series seeks to publish selected works of foremost experts in the field of counselling and psychotherapy. Each volume features the best of a key figure's work, bringing together papers that have been published widely in the professional literature. In this way the work of leading counsellors and psychotherapists is made accessible in single volumes.

Windy Dryden
Series Editor

Titles in the Psychotherapy Series

Foreword

For far too long, psychotherapy was, by and large, available only to a privileged few who lived in metropolitan areas and who could afford private fees. During the last two decades, services for those in need have been created in many parts of the country within the National Health Service. Dr Aveline has been, and remains, a pioneer in that development. This wide-ranging, rich book is an eloquent testimony to his originality of mind, professional skill and personal dedication in pursuing such a demanding, and indeed daunting, task. I owe him a large debt of gratitude, both professionally and personally, for what he gave me during years when we worked together to promote psychotherapy in the Midlands and the north of England.

'Psychotherapy' has become a nebulous term. It covers a babel of tongues which, at best, speak of divergent theories, techniques, and values, and, at worst, become 'sounding brass' and 'tinkling cymbal'. Dr Aveline cuts through much current jargon in an urgently needed attempt to formulate an approach which, in his words, is 'pragmatic, practical and effective'. In stating his personal credo as being both 'romantic' and 'scientific', practical and creative, he uses such ordinary and yet potent words as 'loneliness', 'hope', 'choice' and 'love'. A coherent theory of individual and group therapy, in which the 'corrective emotional experience' here-and-now is central, embodies the basic value of relationships between people.

In the clash between powerful schools of psychotherapy 'eclecticism' becomes a dirty word, dismissed as a feeble mish-mash. It is refreshing to read Mark Aveline's critical advocacy of a standpoint which is open to learning from very different theories and methods, illustrated by his own training and clinical practice. That he practises what he preaches is evident in the Nottingham service and training in which he has sought an 'integrative psychotherapy' holding together therapists of different disciplines with different orientations. Such openness does not imply a lack of a personal viewpoint, and one, among many of the author's interesting, timely and vigorously held opinions, is expressed in his defence of the present unfashionable 'medical model'.

Mark Aveline cares for people. One sentence echoes throughout his papers on theoretical concepts, practical techniques, methods of training and discussions of organisation: 'Psychotherapy is about people as human beings' (see Chapter 1).

Robert F. Hobson
Honorary Reader in Psychotherapy
University of Manchester

Contents

Part II   Group psychotherapy

Part III   Training and supervision

Chapter 15

Chapter 16

Dedication

To my mentors: both those whom I have known – Jerome Frank, Bob Hobson, Heinz Wolff, Jock Sutherland, David Stafford-Clark, Edward Herst, Don Bannister, Millar Mair, Henry Walton, Morris Carstairs and Hans Strupp – and those whom I know only through their writing – Alfred Adler, Karen Horney, Harry Stack Sullivan, Rollo May and Irwin Yalom.

Introduction

A Romantic and a Scientific View

Psychotherapy has been at the centre of my working life for more than 20 years, and as an ideal for much longer. My view of the subject is both romantic and scientific. In any age, but especially in our Western culture which is so driven by technological advance and materialistic self-concern, the unique experience of individuals is important and needs to be attended to. Psychotherapy first and foremost does that. Each of us is unique and none can know exactly what it is like to be the other. But if we pay careful attention to the meaning that the other places upon his or her experience, we can draw on our sufficient similarity and extend a helping and helpful hand to our fellow in need. This is where psychotherapy begins.

My view is romantic because it supposes that there is goodwill in the world and that the constraining legacy of adverse experience in childhood and later in life can be mitigated. Just as in Samuel Johnson's *bon mot* about a man most unhappy in marriage who married again immediately after his wife's death, my therapeutic optimism may be – and sometimes is – the triumph of hope over experience, but to be optimistic at heart is an essential characteristic for a psychotherapist. I am on less romantic ground when I assume as I do that each person makes a contribution to the genesis and maintenance of his or her situation and can legitimately be held responsible for that contribution. Two postulates stem from this position, namely that of personal responsibility for the contribution and the freedom to exercise choice. I accept of course that circumstance and physical endowment may set narrow limits on a person's freedom to act in life. However, the choices a person makes, be they negative or positive, for contraction or expansion, in fear or with courage, shape in no small part his or her future. It is at the point of choice that the psychotherapist makes one of his or her special contributions to the endeavour that is psychotherapy: to help the other take hold of life and become its architect; to move from the role of victim to re-shaper and re-director of a life that is problematic for its owner. Several of the papers in this book address this and the other special contributions of the psychotherapist.

My scientific view stems from my training as a doctor. Medical thinking is deep-rooted in my being. Though I use few of the technical skills of medicine in my day-to-day practice and stand in awe of the ever-expanding complexity of medical knowledge, I think of myself as a doctor and take pride in that status. It is part of my history and what I bring to my work. One legacy of my medical training is an imperative to think clearly and deductively about clinical problems, and, even more so, about the body of knowledge that frames our understanding and justifies interventions. Much of what is said to be known in psychotherapy is actually supposition or the assertion of dogma. In theory at least, I want to know what is the evidence for a piece of theory or the effectiveness of a therapy. The triple evils of lack of time, resource and energy militate against personal evaluation of these questions, except in a minor way: their importance remains beyond dispute. Alarm bells ring for me when others adopt an extreme stance in theory or practice. Reductionism and simplification do not serve our patients well.

The 'Medical Model'

Medical critics are wont to hang round the neck of their villains the epithet 'users of the medical model'. In this model, attention is supposedly only given to the physical aspects of a patient's being, his or her disordered biochemistry and physiology, genetic vulnerability and physical endowment. The person as a person is lost to view under a weight of investigations, technical procedures and invasive therapies with fierce side-effects. Their existence as people who think, feel and hurt is denied, and the importance of the context of their disorder, its meaning, time in life and interaction with family, friends and work are minimised. This is medicine without a soul – all body and no person, all science and no art.

I do not recognise this model and certainly not as one to which to aspire. I do not deny that some doctors are brutally narrow in their focus – indeed it was the experience of seeing some of these men at work that strengthened my resolve to enter psychiatry and try to do better – and I accept that the exigencies of acute medicine may force giving priority to physical aspects of illness. Also the competitiveness of medical life and the force-feeding of facts in medical school encourage an emphasis on what is knowable and tangible. Little value is placed on matters psychological by many doctors and mental disorder is charged with stigma. But this is not, as I understand it, what the medical model is about. The medical model is about holding an open mind about diagnosis and causation, sifting the evidence, considering all the factors – physical, social and psychological – and constructing an appraisal that gives due weight to each. It is to do with seeing the person as a whole, not as pure *soma* or *psyche* but as an interdependent both, and doing your best for both. In psychiatry in the first quarter of the century, Adolf Meyer and, in medicine recently, George Engel, have been leading proponents of the holistic approach. A welcome recognition of this stance is to be found in the 1991 consultation paper from the General Medical Council which states that in medical undergraduate training 'the primary aim . . . is for the student to acquire an understanding of health and disease, and the prevention and management of the latter, in the *context of the whole individual in his or her place in society*' (my italics).

As well as my questioning attitude to received wisdom, my medical model urges me to see multiple elements at work in the genesis of the patient's problems. I use the term 'patient' without apology. Its Latin origin simply means 'one who suffers'. My role and that of other psychotherapists is to attempt to mitigate that suffering though, paradoxically, the greater understanding that can arise through explorative psychotherapy may accentuate suffering and certainly does not smooth away the psychological pain that is inherent in human life. In my understanding, I prefer to start with simple explanations which have surface validity and which address current important interpersonal issues before moving into more speculative deep explanations. My bias is towards a consideration of a person's character in the context of his or her life and the recurrent, self-defeating or maladaptive patterns of interaction that he or she shows. But I also want to have within view his or her physical being, and use the remedy of medication when appropriate.

Pharmacotherapy and psychotherapy are often portrayed as negative opposites: the former driving the real problem underground and the latter unnecessarily stirring up psychological conflicts. Neither position is wholly valid; both approaches have their place. A speedy biological remedy has much to recommend it and may be essential to preserve life in depressive illness, or to raise the patient's ability to think to the point where he or she can participate in explorative psychotherapy. What is important is to be aware of the meaning of prescribing and receiving medication. On the negative side, it may represent a transferential tug into action – a plea for rescue – that would be better analysed than yielded to by the therapist. The therapist may be responding to the patient's fantasy that it is possible to resolve problems passively and without assuming responsibility for the choices that have been made and are being made in that person's life (Aveline, 1991).

Formative Influences

Like most psychotherapists, my path to psychotherapy has been shaped by personal history. My early years were spent in comfortable seclusion with my mother, two aunts, grandmother and great-grandmother, shielded from the upheavals of the Second World War but aware that danger could suddenly come from without. I remember hiding under the kitchen table when the doodlebugs, the German flying bombs, droned overhead, and the spurt of fear when their engines cut out and they began their plummet to earth. My father's return from army service ended this precarious idyll and instituted the move at the age of four from the south coast to London. Now that the war was over, I soon acquired a brother and sister and, like it or not, moved into the character-forming role of the responsible firstborn. Being a dayboy at a local preparatory school, a biggish fish in a little pond, with some specially supportive female teachers, a group of close friends and loving parents, was a pleasant time: my nature expanded. Going to boarding-school, Charterhouse, was a shock and I coped by retreating into myself. A bleak 2 years at the bottom of the pile, made worse by scant food, complex petty rules of conduct that had to be obeyed, the threat of the cane and verbal bullying that I endured rather than fought against, sensitised me to loneliness, sadness and cruelty. I steeled myself to survive, and found friendship outside the preferred order of team and house sports in mountaineering and scouting. Later I enjoyed the enormous diversity of interest and activity that is fostered in the senior part of a great public school.

My choice of career as I came to the end of the sixth form lay between forestry and medicine, both in my view being nurturative occupations that sustained the natural order. I had an idea that I wanted to work in a personal way with people and their emotional difficulties. A general practitioner advised that that was what psychotherapists did but that I would do well to qualify as a doctor first. Despite being critical of the way that medicine can be taught and practised, I am glad that I followed his advice. Medicine gave me a depth of knowledge about the workings of the body that no other training could have provided, and a position of influence that is all important if one wishes to have one's ideas put into practice.

I went to a very traditional medical school, St Bartholomew's in London. I did not mind competing academically and in commitment to the work, but I resented the way that advancement seemed linked to dressing correctly and being a member, often by invitation only, of the right societies, those that were patronised by influential consultants. In the caste system of medicine, psychiatry occupied – as it still does – a lowly position. Teaching was by lecture, lauding the then-amazing advances in psychopharmacology, and by staged demonstrations of the features of major psychotic illness which demeaned both patient and spectator. This experience motivated several of us to enter psychiatry and half of these gravitated to psychotherapy. Medical student life in those days was not dominated as it tends to be now by the inexorable educational process of continuous assessment. I had time to climb and row and drank deep of the culture afforded by London, the cinema, theatre and the visual arts.

After a dalliance with surgery, paediatrics and general practice, I began my psychiatric training at Guy's Hospital. My two consultants were markedly different. David Stafford-Clark, a great showman whose popularising of psychiatry had done much to de-stigmatise the subject, taught me to take a human approach with patients and John Fleminger, a man no less concerned with his patients than 'D S-C', reminded me of their physical being. Work in liaison psychiatry further developed an abiding interest in the vicissitudes of human experience and the inter-play with personal vulnerability. In terms of psychotherapy, I was fast becoming a mongrel – and all the better for that! My supervisors were of humanistic, Jungian and behavioural persuasions.

After 3 years, my wife and I moved to Edinburgh, where I had been appointed senior registrar. Edinburgh was a breath of fresh air after London where the organic model of psychiatry was too dominant for my taste. Under the inspiring leadership of Morris Carstairs, the Royal Edinburgh Hospital buzzed with the diverse voices of experts in social psychiatry, psychoanalysis, epidemiology, parasuicide, neuropharma-cology and sleep disorders. I was impressed that such difference could be contained within a single institution, just as I am appalled by the present tendency to split dynamic from cognitive–behavioural psycho-therapy, a process which will surely impoverish both if they fail to learn from each other's strengths. Morris Carstairs' will to maintain the Edinburgh tradition of pluralism was one potent factor in its success; another, more structural, factor was employing senior staff who were well informed about approaches other than their own, and who had sufficient space and facilities to develop their specialisms.

I spent most of my time working for Henry Walton on the in-patient ward that he directed, and in liaison psychiatry at the Western General Hospital. Ward 1 provided intense psychoanalytically oriented therapy in individual, group and milieu forms for patients with personality dis-order and psychiatric illness. Some patients' admission lasted upwards of a year. For the patients and for me, it was an intense, absorbing experience; all who immersed themselves were changed. In addition, I had a great deal of training in group therapy from Jock Sutherland, who had recently retired from being Director of the Tavistock Clinic. From Jock, I gained a keen appreciation of the importance of process in groups. Experiences gained mainly outside the hospital in encounter, psychodrama and art therapy fostered the conviction that the fulcrum for personal change rests with 'here-and-now' relationships. I learnt that being a member of a cohesive, purposeful therapy group can be a uniquely encouraging experience in a person's life, offering as it does a rare opportunity for altruism and unlimited scope for interpersonal learning.

Nottingham

Come 1974 and I was ready to put my ideals and ideas into practice. I was appointed to a new post in Nottingham, with seven sessions to develop psychotherapy service and training and four to oversee a long-stay day-hospital. In the day-hospital, the introduction of groups and the fostering of personal autonomy and social interdependence led, over 5 years, to a halving of numbers attending, and opened the way to my formally becoming full-time in psychotherapy.

The penultimate paper in this volume describes how the Nottingham Psychotherapy Unit has developed. Nottingham had the priceless advantage to my way of thinking of there being no set pattern of NHS psychotherapy service to constrain my efforts. A compact Midlands city, sustained by light industry, and a university whose new medical school was attracting an influx of talented colleagues, located sufficiently close to London to be in touch with colleagues there but sufficiently far away not to be under their thumb, seemed an excellent place to build up a service that was dedicated to providing appropriate psychotherapy without fee through the NHS. I have to write 'was', as the new imperatives of cost, charging for service and active management introduce a changed order in the NHS that may fundamentally alter our service.

To date, my energies have been directed to developing a range of effective psychotherapies, suitable for NHS practice: teaching the necessary skills at undergraduate, post-qualification and specialist levels; establishing a Department of Psychotherapy with sufficient skilled staff to (1) provide a specialist service for the more disturbed patient and (2) staff the training programme; researching the subject; contributing to the literature; and playing a part in the development of a forward-looking specialty of psychiatry, both locally and nationally.

For the first 5 years of my appointment, I was the only Consultant Psychotherapist in the Trent Health Region. Now there are companion Departments of Psychotherapy in Leicester (1979), Derby (1980) and Lincoln (1985). In Nottingham, the Department has grown to two consultants (the second consultant being appointed in 1987) and 12 full-time specialist psychotherapists, drawn from all the health care professions, and covering both dynamic and cognitive–behavioural psychotherapy.

Skill as a psychotherapist is not the preserve of any one profession. In staffing the department, I have created career opportunities for talented therapists from all the mental health care professions and charged each member of staff with special responsibility for developing the psychotherapeutic skills of their profession of origin. A recent initiative is the establishment of adult psychotherapist posts, an as yet ad hoc grade within the NHS, which has the advantage of broadening the recruitment pool and providing a better career ladder for some. My aim has been to bring together within a single department therapists with diverse orientations, and to provide a setting where essential differences can be preserved and learning from the strengths of each approach promoted. This provides the optimum setting for matching therapy to patient need, and to have available the range of skills necessary to support an extensive training programme.

Life as a Psychotherapist

What has the work in Nottingham been like for me? In the beginning, as consultant, I was the flag-carrier for the specialty of psychotherapy and its standard-keeper. Now these functions are also carried by all the psychotherapists in the department. There has been much administration, and long battles to get posts established and grades improved. Training schemes such as the South Trent Training in Dynamic Psychotherapy, a specialist training within the NHS collaboratively mounted by the departments in Nottingham, Leicester, Derby and Lincoln, have evolved over the years and required endless hours of negotiation. There has been work in London in committee and at conference to put psychotherapy outside London on the map. If I had my time again, I would not have wanted to miss out on building something new that I believe in, and on testing my strength, but now some of the arguments have lost their freshness.

As a psychotherapist, I hope that the psychotherapy that like-minded colleagues and I provide is pragmatic, practical and effective. My particular interest is in group and focal therapy, emphasising interpersonal, humanistic and existential concerns.

Practising psychotherapy is a demanding occupation. But it also allows me to give of my best. In concentrating on my patient's concerns, I am at my least self-full. I can bring to bear my tenacity and patience in seeing the endeavour through to some resolution. I can convey my solidarity with the other in need, and share my understanding of what it is to be that person. I can try to help and not exploit the other's vulnerability.

In entering into many lives as a therapist and assisting change, there is privilege and hardship. In these entered lives, there is much sadness and tragedy and the remnant of hope that has nearly been battered to death. When one thinks of the world as it is, with so much injustice, cruelty and ill-fortune, it is impossible not to feel saddened; in therapy, one is confronted with this at first hand. I cannot see that therapy can succeed unless the therapist cares about what is happening in the patient's life and is open to feeling what the other is feeling. Thus, in the course of the week, one is pulled hither and thither in sadness, frustration, anger and loss, and in the service of completing the very self-handicapping patterns of interaction that are the essence of the other person's difficulty in relationships. Of course there are times of success and shared pleasure in achievement but, for every two steps forward, there is at least one step backward. Each person's defences have been developed for good reasons and are not lightly given up. There is, as it were, a hidden pressing invitation from the patient to be drawn into their relationship pattern and arrive at the old sad end of failed interaction, and to see only the offered negative self and not the hidden, more able, self. Living with all this and the fact that what one has done may not be enough to takes its toll.

In taking on the role of psychotherapist, one opens oneself to change and the loss of personal illusions. The encounter of therapy changes both patient and therapist. Through seeing oneself more clearly, a ripple of adjustment and readjustment is set going in both lives. Some emotional growth follows. However, I have noticed a constriction in my expressive self as I settle yet further into the Sullivanian participant observer role of therapist. Years of being there for the patient, of reflecting rather than initiating and of leaving space for the other to make decisions, has exacerbated a passive aspect of myself which is curious to see how events will fall without my shaping. I have become too good at hearing sadness and anger and, in ordinary life, find myself automatically drawing others out rather than pressing my view. I find I need to have variety in what I do each day. Planning, writing, committee work and, to a lesser extent, supervision, allow me to express my more assertive, decisive self, without which I would be off-balance; I look also to the physical activities of tennis, walking, gardening and bonfire-making as essential correctives. To guard against a false sense of superiority, I need the challenge of ordinary interactions far away from the protected world of therapy. Though I regret some decisions and moves not made, I would not change the broad direction of my life. I remain an optimistic idealist and intend to go on contributing to the field of psychotherapy.

Selection of Papers

In making the selection for this volume, I thank Windy Dryden for his guidance. Research papers and those of limited general interest have not been included. Instead three themes have been addressed:

1. What is psychotherapy?
2. How may one practise group psychotherapy to good effect?
3. Issues in training in individual and group psychotherapy and the provision of service in the NHS.

Reference

AVELINE, M. (1991). Anxiety and stress-related disorders. In: J. Holmes (Ed.), *Psychotherapy in Psychiatric Practice*. Edinburgh: Churchill Livingstone.

Part I
Psychotherapy

I make no claim for deep originality in the five papers in this section. They are, however, the fruit of hard-won experience, and chart my progress in elaborating what is central to effective psychotherapy.

The first paper 'Towards a conceptual framework of psychotherapy – a personal view' is by way of a personal credo. I have always found that the exercise of writing down what I think helps me define what I think; this is my original and most systematic attempt. Psychotherapy is about people as human beings, and their capacity to form good relationships. In the process of therapy (and of living), the key elements are hope, trust, sensitivity, responsibility, risk, personal meaning, choice and freedom. The issues are commonplace: loneliness, rejection, acceptance, love, self-doubt, and fears of being overwhelmed and constrained. I use these ordinary words because of their very ordinariness and to supplant technical language that mystifies, alienates or distances. Were I to rewrite this paper, I would want to stress the importance of humour, enjoyment and affirmation in therapy, and that the long list of desirable characteristics in the therapist points to an ideal that no one person achieves.

Alexander and French's 'corrective emotional experience' may prove to be a central unifying concept in psychotherapy. There is a potential for personal change at times of tension in the encounter of therapy ('The process of being known and the initiation of change') when the therapist is being drawn into the patient's problematic and self-limiting patterns of interaction. The challenge for the therapist is to relate to the person as he or she is, and to the hidden, more able, self that is emergent ('The provision of illusion in psychotherapy'). However through the invitation exerted by transference and the prompting of countertransference, it is all too easy to end up recreating the traumas of the past and reinforcing the maladaptive patterns of the present. 'Parameters of danger: interactive elements in the therapy

1

dyad' outlines how, in Nottingham, we prepare trainees for such hap-penings and, more speculatively, have tried to select pairings of patient and therapist that promise well for the encounter of therapy.

1990 saw the appointment of the first Professor of Psychotherapy in a British University, namely at Warwick. This was a long-awaited event: psychotherapy has been neglected by British academics, who have been sceptical about its value as a therapy and its status as a research-able subject. With a few notable exceptions, psychotherapists at the dynamic end of the spectrum have not helped by being reluctant to open their consulting rooms to critical but potentially constructive research enquiry. Whilst fully recognising the great difficulties in con-ducting meaningful research, I hope that the subject will be refined through the enquiring, scholarly and non-doctrinaire approach that academic departments could provide. 'Psychotherapy: a fundamental discipline but an academic orphan' expresses this ideal.

Chapter 1
Towards a Conceptual Framework of Psychotherapy: A Personal View

In the columns of this journal last year Miller Mair (1977) advocated the development of a personal psychology that took its origin from questions of vital import to the proponent. By beginning with personal experience it is possible to reach concepts of relevance and importance in ordinary life, and not be side-tracked into subordinating relevance to simplification in order to satisfy the rigorous demands of scientific method. This paper takes up the invitation issued by Mair. Over the last decade as a psychotherapist and psychiatrist I have sought to question what I am doing in therapy and why I am doing it. Some answers have emerged from my work only to raise further questions, and each question and each answer parallel similar enquiries I make of myself living my own life. The two dimensions of work and existence overlap, coincide, diverge and illuminate each other. The practice of psychotherapy requires the verification of everyday life and must arise naturally out of the personality of the therapist. In this endeavour work and our own existence cannot be divorced. Harmony between the two enriches both.

To promote debate and clarify my own thinking I wish to set down my present views. To some the views may seem self-evident and to others heretical. For myself they represent an evolution in which many models have been tried and their better features retained, but which I do not regard as having reached the end-point. To date, my psychological mentors, in order of exposure, have advocated a humanistic, behavioural, Jungian, personal construct, Freudian, developmental, encounter and gestalt, object relations, systems theory, social network, vector, Rogerian, interpersonal and existential approach. For many years I have been interested in ethics, moral philosophy and the

From M.O. Aveline (1979). Towards a conceptual framework of psychotherapy – a personal view. *British Journal of Medical Psychology*, **52**, 271–275, with permission.

insights that various religions have into the nature of humankind and the purpose of life. Flesh has been given to these constructions through enperiences in living, through learning of the lives of others and in literature, poems, plays and paintings. The validity of these constructions has been judged against their familiarity in everyday life. From this eclectic abundance, what remains?

Psychotherapy is about people as human beings. This fundamental assumption, which drew me to medicine in the beginning, may be regarded as being so obvious that it does not need stating, but yet, if not asserted, it all too easily becomes lost in the face of technology, reductionism and blinkered vision. Psychotherapy is not exclusively to do with patients and certainly it is antithetical to the view of the person as a small or non-existent appendage to the patient's illness. Psychotherapy is concerned with the problems that people have in living their lives and in living with each other. Although symptoms often have meaning and illnesses psychodynamic significance, I feel that psychotherapy has less to offer in elucidating those meanings and significance than in attending to human relations, the ways in which a person or people can and do live. The focus of psychotherapy is the contribution that the individual or individuals in the context of their circumstances make to the problem or difficulty. The colloquial phrase 'life is what you make it' has special importance for pyschotherapists. The justification for psychotherapy is personal change – change in the aspect of life that has the potential to be under one's control. One's position in life is determined by oneself, by chance and by circumstance. Under circumstance I include the people and physical reality that constitute one's context and also one's physical being, both constitutional endowment and temporal stage in life. A woman past the age of child-bearing cannot conceive, a man with one leg will never run 100 yards in 10 seconds, a man with a strong sense of duty and many responsibilities cannot abandon them without experiencing guilt, and the cultivation of certain aspects of self may be incompatible with continuing to live in one's usual community. To suggest otherwise is ludicrous and unfair. If nothing else, psychotherapy must be responsible.

However, with the caveat that chance and circumstance are equal determinants of what a person can do, my psychotherapy assumes that people are responsible for their lives and have choice. This assumption is uncomfortable for many. The stark and, at times, bleak realism that this implies prepares the individual for action on his or her own behalf and does not allow him or her to take cover behind the determinism of the past.

As human beings we act upon the meaning of our experience. Unlike lesser animals, we are able to think, and this ability confers upon us the freedom to decide. Our decisions are based upon the remembrances of previous similar experiences, their outcome, their consequences for good and bad, our perception of the present experience and our anticipation of the various futures that could follow. Humans cannot make context-free and history-free assessments. All personal experience has meaning, the current meaning being shaped by past meaning and the present and future consequences. As Sir Dennis Hill (1970) has pointed out, biological science is concerned with mechanism or 'how' things happen, whereas understanding human nature is concerned with meaning, with the 'whys' of human behaviour. Psychotherapy is about the latter and has something valid to say about human relationships. It follows that the main focus of psychotherapy should be on the real or anticipated interactions with others. We are not Plato's men chained to see only shadows of the real world. We can face what is. The perspective is now and the future and the past only in so far as it frees the individual from it.

Classical psychoanalysis has emphasised the deterministic pattern set down in the first few years of life (S. Freud) or even the first few months (M. Klein) so much so that *all* interaction between therapist and patient (i.e. one who suffers) would be scrutinised for unconscious significance transferred from the past. Shifting the focus from 'then and there' to 'here and now' and 'tomorrow' transmutes the hallowed questions of psychoanalysis. 'What is the meaning of the symptom?' becomes 'What problems does he have as a person?' 'Who am I to the patient?' becomes 'How do I feel about him?' and 'How does he feel about me?' 'In what ways is he tied to the past?' becomes 'What possible futures may he make for himself?' The priority of a relatively apersonal provision of insight leading to the release from the bonds with the past is demoted in favour of an active replanning of now and tomorrow. One might almost say that the feature that distinguishes patients from non-patients is that the former have an inflexible and limited variety of ways of perceiving their experience and acting on it. Karen Horney (1939) termed this 'rigidity in reaction'. Successful psychotherapy enables the individual to develop for him- or herself new and alternative strategies for personally difficult situations. Psychotherapy must attend to life as it is, and help people to be more free to act. In this I see psychotherapy being a practical discipline and not an excuse for abstraction or an invitation to become a way of life.

In order to communicate we need words and concepts, but I find that the language of human nature as used in scientific journals frequently fails the tests of humanity and comprehensibility. The issues of psychotherapy are commonplace. They include the feelings of loneliness, rejection, acceptance, love, self-doubt, and fears of being overwhelmed, unable and constrained. It is a reflection of how far we in psychiatry have moved from what Kathleen Jones (1978) has termed

'the natural stance of Psychiatry, straddling social science and medicine' that these everyday and important concepts are not given formal
recognition in our major textbooks, and would by some be denied to
fall within the province of psychiatrists.

How may personal change come about? Commonly people enter
therapy demoralised by their experience of life and lacking in sufficient
trust in others to allow their relationships to improve. It is the first task
of therapy to rediscover hope, the common ingredient of all healing
processes (Frank, 1973). The second task is to redevelop the capacity
to trust. The medium for all this is the human exchange between
patient and therapist, the words, the ideas, the reactions and feelings. I
know that when I am with people whom I trust and whom I feel like
me, I am more open, expansive, more fully myself. When I am less sure
about those about me, I am constrained and cautious. So it is in therapy.
Before people can become free to act on life as it is for them, they must
build up trust in the setting of their own therapy. Trust cannot be
imposed and has to be earned through being trustworthy in some issue
of personal importance. Here the personal qualities of the therapist are
all important, not only in meeting the challenge of a test of trust but in
providing a sufficiently secure background so that the individual can
work on increasing self-awareness, awareness of others, perceiving the
consequences of his actions, reducing inner conflicts, correcting misperceptions and taking the risk of living more fully. Honesty and reality
are tempered with optimism. Change arises through encountering
one's context and transcending previous patterns and strategies, or at
least consciously choosing to remain as one is. The history of psychotherapy is muddied by the conflict between the early writers who gave
their accolade to thought and the provision of insight, and the later
behaviourists who emphasised action. The middle ground of the
quality of relationship between therapist and patient has long been
recognised and is increasingly accepted by both extremes. The truth
must lie in a judicious mixture of all three, as they are all facets of being
a human being.

By taking as my perspective 'now' and 'the future', I do not mean to
decry the importance of the past. Indeed it may be crucial that the
therapist is aware of what past influences are currently operating in the
patient *and* in him- or herself, but this is attending to the past only in so
far as it is necessary, and not making it the be-all of therapy. After all,
we go through life enjoying our days and anticipating our tomorrows
and not sitting on the van of time looking backwards.

The assertion that psychotherapy is either thought or action is a
travesty of a complex truth; similarly, abstracting people from their
social context and interviewing them in the consulting room may make
for ease of comprehension, but this simplification often excludes the

very factors that are vital to attend to if change is to occur successfully. Although sooner or later the therapeutic relationship will mirror the problematic attitudes or behaviour that the patient has in his or her real life, work with a therapist separate from that life introduces an extra stage in reaping the benefit of his or her endeavours. Benefit achieved when working directly with the natural context of the patient is immediate and relevant. As a rule of thumb, when an individual's problem involves named people within their context then I work with that natural grouping, but if the problem is one of general social relationships, then a group is an appropriate medium, and if the individual's problems are essentially those of his or her relationship with him- or herself or if a period of preparation is needed, I suggest one-to-one therapy.

In this encounter between therapist and patient both must be able to feel, think and act. The personal attributes that qualify the therapist for his or her role include patience, persistence, passion, integrity, imagination, sensitivity and optimism about people. He or she must possess the ability to pass the desperation point and not give up in the face of seeming disasters. At the moment of crisis when all hangs in the balance, to continue is difficult but essential if new learning is to occur. The meaning of such a success is strong and clear. It is obvious that the therapist must possess a desire for the well-being of others. In my view, these qualities can only come about through having a good experience of life, though not such a perfect one as to insulate one from frustration and anxiety, the experience of which is essential in the empathic understanding of another. Jung (1967) remarked that 'only the wounded physician heals'. The therapist needs a strong sense of his or her own identity and, at times, an instinct for survival. This fallibly human and yet super-human being must have both confidence in what he or she is doing and humility about his or her limitations.

Human beings have always busied themselves in making order out of chaos. The notion that there are rules to be discovered in the process of living is seductive, but the student of life soon learns that what is right for one person is wrong for another, and that what is right for one now may not be so tomorrow. The pre-eminence of trust, cooperation and sufficient independence in good personal relationships does not alter, but the psychotherapist has to face the fact that the paradoxes of life are inherent in his or her work. The therapist will do different things with different people, and with the same person at different times. Besides being trustworthy, hopeful and sharing, he or she may be flexible and firm, gentle and tough, accepting and discriminating. Giving advice, setting tasks and intervening are seen by purists as stultifying to others' striving for maturity, but may be the correct thing to do when the other is bemused by options and needs to act, or is about to fail in a tragic, self-limiting way. Equally, to live the lives of others for them is to render them children, and to dictate how they should live is presumptuous. (Not to be aware of one's own views is dangerous ignorance!) The path between cocooning and irresponsible exposure is narrow; in treading it, the therapist has the advantage of not being the other, of being able to choose what to say and when, and the responsibility of trying to see what may happen. These are the qualities of a sense of timing and clear sight. The wish to abate the psychological pain inherent in living may cloud the vision of the therapist as to what is right for a fellow traveller. One's own solutions are not so wonderful, and compassion for those of others is important, as is the ability to let others lead their own lives. In this sense, my psychotherapy is not bombastic or intrusive, but neither is it soft and passive.

Our way of leading our lives is perfused by the view of the world that we have. We cannot bury our heads in the sand and ignore the consequences of our actions or what we help others to achieve. Therapists are not technicians passively working at the direction of another. They cannot evade their ethical responsibility or deny their moral beliefs (although they must guard against imposing them inappropriately). A constant dilemma is the balance between the needs of the individual and of his or her community. In its practice, psychotherapy is not and never should be context-free or culture-free.

My conception of psychotherapy is that it is a practical discipline and a creative art; certainly it is hard work. Each person demands an individual approach in which one hopes to create space for manoeuvre in the inner world of meaning and in the external world of context. I recognise that there are many dimensions and purposes in life, and try to guard against reductionism and also approaches that are demeaning or trivialising. I expect to be involved in a two-way process or conversation in which, although the need is with the person, both of us may be changed or 'stretched'. We are engaged upon the same journey. I hope that the relationship will be genuine, equal in feeling, asymmetrical in disclosure (R. Hobson, 1977, personal communication). My acceptance of the other will not be bland and total but discriminating, because this parallels ordinary life, promotes learning and allows me more freedom to react. The setting – individual, natural or artificial group – and the ploys – role rehearsal, psychodrama, projective techniques – may vary. The recurrent element is the relationship and the ideas and practical effects that arise out of it. To write all this is much simpler than to practise, which often seems confusing, unsure, impossible and exhilarating. Yet to attempt therapy is a fundamentally important human activity and, in my view, psychiatry is a non-discipline without it.

The key words for me in this paper are hope, trust, sensitivity, responsibility, risk, choice and freedom. They imply a certain view of humankind that is personally important, and reflect my belief that psychotherapy is concerned with the human capacity to form good relationships. Crucial though it is, this is only one aspect of human beings, and so psychotherapy has to take its place alongside the mechanical, intellectual and spiritual aspects of existence. It will be clear that the qualities I regard as being important in the therapist reside in the individual, not in any one profession, and are capable of development and training only if already present. The quantities themselves are ideals which are not possessed by any one person all the time.

I conclude by offering a definition of a psychotherapist. A psychotherapist is a person who is professionally committed to helping others fulfil their human potential for good personal relationships. His or her belief in this potential will be grounded in his or her experience of life and in practising the art of psychotherapy. His or her ability to help derives from his or her personal qualities and knowledge, which will have been developed through practice, supervision and becoming skilled in a variety of approaches and settings.

References

FRANK, J.D. (1973). *Persuasion and Healing*, 2nd edn. Baltimore, MD: Johns Hopkins University Press.

HILL, D. (1970). On the contribution of psychoanalysis to psychiatry. *British Journal of Psychiatry* **117**, 609–115.

HORNEY, K. (1939). *New Ways in Psychoanalysis*. London: Routledge & Kegan Paul.

JONES, K. (1978). Society looks at the psychiatrist. *British Journal of Psychiatry* **132**, 321–332.

JUNG, C.G. (1967). *Memories, Dreams, Reflections*. London: Fontana.

MAIR, J.M. (1977). Psychology and psychotherapy: Some common concerns. *British Journal of Medical Psychology* **50**, 21–25.

Chapter 2
The Process of Being Known and the Initiation of Change

Prior Theory and Practice

The life of a psychotherapist may be likened to a journey without end. The way is shaped by where one starts from, who walked with you in the early stages, what persons, patients, friends and foes are encountered, and whether the terrain is harsh or easy going. Along the way there are many unforeseen twists and turns, doubling-backs and advances. Some divides in the path lead to dead ends, others to vantage points whence new vistas can be seen. Often, only in retrospect can one see why this path was chosen and not that. In a lifetime, only part of the great country of human life can be explored. To reach some point of rest is comfortable; to continue exploring is to know strange things and to be humble before the vastness of what is to be known. Quite soon, one discovers that others – therapists, poets, writers and philosophers – have explored the same domain and described what seems new. And yet, travellers' tales mean little till one has journeyed to the point where discovery lies. The psychotherapies that I describe in this chapter were two such journeys.

In 18 years as a psychotherapist, 7 of these as a trainee and 11 as a consultant, I have worked with many patients and read widely. Sometimes I feel that I have learnt a great deal, but often that I have hardly begun.

My path to psychotherapy has been unusually broad. I have been supervised by humanistic, Jungian and behavioural therapists and have been influenced by seeing the application of personal construct theory in therapy. I have worked on an intensive in-patient unit with a Freudian developmental perspective, and have learnt the skills of leadership

From M.O. Aveline (1988). The process of being known and the initiation of change. In W. Dryden (Ed.), *Key Cases in Psychotherapy*, Croom-Helm, London, with permission.

of a closed group from an object-relations supervisor versed in the works of Fairbairn and Guntrip. Another perspective in my learning was opened up by personal experience in encounter groups and the use of creative therapies. Latterly, I have been impressed by the insights and the way of working developed in the cultural, interpersonal and existential schools. From all this comes a way of practising psychotherapy that is still evolving, and a conclusion that there is no royal road in psychotherapy. All approaches illuminate aspects of any one condition; none is a total answer; each will appeal differentially to patient and therapist.

The unique feature of psychotherapy is the structured professional relationship between the therapist and one or more patients (the word 'patient' is used in the non-pejorative sense of meaning a person who suffers), who meet in a relationship which is genuine, equal in feeling but asymmetrical in disclosure (Hobson, 1985), and which is directed towards assisting the patient in making changes in personal functioning. In this relationship, although the declared need is with one, both may be changed – not shrunk but stretched! The good quality of the relationship restores hope and redevelops trust; it is both the means of change and the substrate for the risky business of developing new strategies for personally difficult situations. In a mechanistic and materialistic world, the deliberate focus on experience and the personal meaning placed upon it asserts the value of that realm of human life. In my therapy, the emphasis on personal responsibility and choice, on what the person can do today and tomorrow rather than on what was done in time gone by, points to change in that portion of the external world that is, or potentially is, under that person's control. The justification for psychotherapy lies in the help that it can provide with the problems that people have in living their lives and living with each other. In this, psychotherapy is a practical discipline and a creative art (Chapter 1).

My differential learning has given a special cast to my practice. In order to highlight changes in my practice from then to now and to contrast with other approaches described in this volume, I will summarise my practice points more dogmatically than is my wont. The importance of the process of being known and the personal history of the therapist – my last two practice points (8 and 9) – was highlighted for me by my key case.

Practice point 1: Countering demoralisation and enhancing hope

Most people seeking psychotherapeutic help are demoralised; their demoralisation results in distress and disability and stems from a sense of failure or of powerlessness to alter themselves and their environment. All types of successful psychotherapy have measures to restore self-confidence and to promote a sense of mastery through successful experiences (Frank, 1973; Aveline, 1984). I actively seek to counter the demoralisation and promote mastery.

Practice point 2: An interpersonal focus

I conceptualise personality as the meeting place of relationships, and all personal disturbance as occurring in or being a function of interpersonal processes. In this, I follow in the footsteps of Adler (1924), Horney (1945) and Sullivan (1953). For me, the individual is not an isolated, static unit but a person who can only properly be seen in the light of his or her actions and the reactions of his or her environment. Whereas much of the work of psychotherapy is to do with elucidating intrapsychic processes, what happens between people is, in my view, the arena in which psychotherapy has most to offer. This arises naturally from the nature of psychotherapy which essentially is a personal remedy for problems of relationship.

Practice point 3: The present is accessible and relevant; the past is less knowable

All memories are distorted by active and passive forgetting, wishful thinking and the selective effect of the context in which they are being retold. In the dyad of patient and therapist, isolated as it usually is from the past and present external social systems, stories are told which can all too easily be assumed to be historically true rather than narratively true. A cosy blaming of faults on to others, and especially parents, may occur, thereby absolving the patient from his or her existential responsibility. What is more knowable and more relevant is what is happening now in the person's life. This is not to say that I am not interested in the past, but only as a prelude to the present and the future.

Practice point 4: Being and becoming

All of us who are psychologically alive are fundamentally involved in the process of being and becoming. We are our 'being in the world', the *Dasein* of Heidegger (1962) and Binswanger (1956), and this being is made up of acts. Acts are more than behaviours; they are intentional steps on the paths that we map for ourselves. As a therapist, I am thus concerned with how the details of interactional sequences in current conflictual relationships both define that person's problematic 'being in the world' and lay down the benchmarks against which change can be determined and significant advances made. It is for difficulties in that world that the patient is seeking help, and it is by change in that world that I judge the success of our mutual endeavour. Hitherto change outside the therapy room was more important for me than change within the room.

Practice point 5: A corrective emotional experience

At some stage, in order to change, the patient has to face his personally most difficult situations and live through them to more fruitful ways of being. The skill of the therapist lies in his or her ability to assist the patient in writing a new end to an old, sad story. In this, it does not particularly matter whether the change occurs inside or outside the therapy situation, and indeed the direct benefit of the latter has obvious advantages (Alexander and French, 1946; Aveline, 1986). Times of crisis in a person's life are particularly potent moments for change. As these cases taught me, continuing the therapy when all hangs in the balance is to take the path that leads to new learning.

In contrast to a purely psychoanalytic model, in my therapy the transferential elements have been background to the focus on current problematic actual relationships. Naturally and usefully, when the outside problematic pattern of interaction is recreated in the therapy relationship, I attend to this, but I do not primarily intend, as a psychoanalyst would, to create that pattern in a transference neurosis. My temperament is not suited to deep regressive work; my assessment of how therapy achieves its ends has not convinced me that it is generally necessary. Progression, not regression, is my motto.

Practice point 6: Significant acts

Each of us develops out of our experience an internal map of how the world is. Each map is different although the landscape is part of the common world; the perspective is determined by individual assumptions. The map enables us to predict our behaviour and that of others, and foresee the outcome of our actions. Frank (1973) aptly terms this 'the assumptive world'. I find the concept straightforward and one that is easily accessible to me and the patient. Ultimately it is through acts, both the acts we do and the ones we do not do, that our assumptive world is reinforced or altered. In my practice, I place great emphasis on comprehending in detail the sequence of interpersonal events in any current problematic situation. I listen for metaphors or images which will form a personal shorthand for significant events or ways of perceiving self. This analysis informs both the patient and me as to what is habitually done, and what would be significant acts of change. Such significant acts may appear relatively unimportant to an uninformed external assessor, but to us they have dynamic importance and, once succeeded in, represent the yielding of those dynamics.

Practice point 7: The indivisibility of the intrapsychic and the interpersonal

Often, psychotherapy writers have emphasised the intrapsychic or the interpersonal to the exclusion of the other, and have likewise addressed their interventions to one and not the other. I see no special priority. The two are indivisible; each reflects and influences the other. When I intervene in the interpersonal world, my exploration takes me straight into the intrapsychic world of meaning. When I intervene in the intrapsychic world, I influence the interpersonal.

Practice point 8: Being known

A *sine qua non* of therapy that extends over time and explicates meaning and experience is a coming together of two explorers: patient and therapist. How they combine is a function of what they explore and who they are as people. Most often the union is not achieved easily. The growing closeness of the union activates in the exchange of therapy the conflicts that stymie the patient in his or her interpersonal life. The emphasis here is on the existential process of being known by another, and less on the transference distortions that regulate that process. This factor was brought into sharp focus by the cases that I describe.

Practice point 9: The personal history of the therapist

In therapy we listen carefully to all that the patient says, but in attempting to make imaginative leaps into his world, to experience the other side (Buber, 1958), we often project on to him or her what we know best – our own determining myths and fantasies. Some might argue that it is impossible to do otherwise. Our own sensitivities enable us to respond to some hurts or outrages better than others. In this key case, aspects of my nature worked for and against the finding of the therapeutic way. I know myself to be tenacious, ambitious and seemingly self-contained; I enjoy creating. I believe myself to be trustworthy. I have a strong reparative element in my make-up and easily feel responsible and guilty. I dislike causing others humiliation or shame. I am acutely aware of anger, especially when it is directed towards me, and am sensitive to movements that others make towards and away from me.

Description of the Key Case

My basic training is in medicine and psychiatry. I work as a consultant psychotherapist in the National Health Service in Britain. My clinical practice is mostly with individual patients seen weekly for usually between 25 and 100 sessions. I also lead therapy groups and spend a small amount of time on marital and family work. I meet with individual patients in my personal office, which is located in an informally furnished house. Patients have a choice of identical armchairs, and sessions are 40 minutes long at the same time each week.

I met with Mary 73 times over a 2½-year period, some time in the last 6 years. Some details of her biography have been altered to preserve confidentiality. In her early thirties, she was living alone and was in the first year of a 3-year vocational training. Four years before, she had broken away from an unhappy marriage, and 6 months before I met her had suffered the major blow of her 5-year-old daughter choosing to go from her to live with her former husband, himself resident 200 miles away.

In her pre-assessmet interview goals in psychotherapy questionnaire, which all referrals to my Unit routinely complete (Aveline and Smith, 1986), she identified as her chief problems depression, a past full of unsuccessful relationships, and feelings of panic when she could no longer maintain a façade of normality. Her life felt futile and without purpose. She felt unable to do what she wanted and to assert her point of view without seeming aggressive. She was plagued by her need to justify herself and a tendency to feel guilty. Perhaps most important of all was her sense of being controlled by events rather than being in control of them and the way in which she had chosen loneliness as a means of self-protection. She wanted to be more positive about life and to overcome her fear of getting close to others and of letting them get close to her.

In working with her, these issues were our focus in considering her outside life, but also became the substance of our exchange within the sessions. On looking back at the therapy, I feel again her sadness, the sudden days and weeks of uplifting hope, and then of bitter disappointment. I remember hesitant approaches to one another and my uncomfortable feelings of being not the person that she required and of having injured her, and then having to repair the damage by making peace. Later the strength was found to overcome these hesitancies, truths were spoken, and the process of change was initiated.

The bare bones of her history as related at the assessment interview with a colleague were of growing up in a family where individuality and the open expression of feeling were not encouraged, especially not by her mother. Her single sibling, a brother 4 years older, conformed and was approved; she did not and was not. Having failed to get into university through not passing one of her 'A' levels, she followed her mother's choice of what was suitable for a girl by taking secretarial training and, then, quickly, marrying. She had little in common with her husband and, despite trying to cement the relationship by having a child, they drifted apart. She emerged from the marriage and – to her great credit – had for 2 or 3 years before she came into therapy held down a demanding job and maintained herself and her daughter. She then took her individuation one step further by beginning post-vocational training; in her class she found herself a decade older than most of her fellow students.

Beginning

The first few sessions contained the key themes, although their significance was not fully apparent to me then. At the first session she observed me with care if not with caution, was forceful in wanting me to tell her what to focus on, and at the same time conveyed the high standard she had for herself and, by implication, had for others. The loss of her daughter to her former husband was a 'kick in the teeth' but not something that she could be angry about as it was one of her principles in life that everyone should make their own decisions; furthermore it was improper for one person to hold on to another. She was hesitant about committing herself to therapy but wanted the weekly session to begin sooner than I could offer.

She felt bitterly alone. Her life was her responsibility, but yet it seemed pointless and empty. Two years before, one important boyfriend, Terry, had wanted her but not her daughter; another, Martin, had wanted her on any terms but she had recoiled from his dependence, which she saw as weakness. To her detriment, she was over-ready to see the point of view of others and to be giving; others, therefore, only saw her competent self. She reacted angrily against my suggestion that this competent self was not just imposed by others but also by herself as a way of avoiding being hurt. She was, she argued, society's victim through its taboo on the expression of sadness and needs. Later, she was to say 'smile and the world laughs with you; cry and you cry alone'.

Sessions 4–9 illustrate aspects of our relationship which were to be writ large later on. Mary had spoken with distaste of her parents' repeated message that they had only stayed together for the children. But facing them with her anger would not be fair and would kill them. I fed back my impression of her being fair on the outside, valuing integrity, and angry and critical inside. My words were an invitation to bring our paths closer together, and for a moment she accepted. She described herself as the 'cuckoo in the family nest', the only one who was different, the one who would not conform to the traditional female role. With approval in my voice, I emphasised that, for her, being different was life-saving, but that she had paid and was paying the price of hostility and misunderstanding by others. She picked up my encouragement to take risks, to try relationships again, and retreated – perhaps I had been coercive – crying that she did not want to be hurt again. I criticised myself for running ahead.

A black cloud had descended by the next week and I deserved her anger for suggesting that her state was related to the week before. In addition, in her eyes, I was inhuman, cool and detached whereas she was human and full of feelings; to show these to me would be humiliating. Suicide was one solution, better than her previous escape routes of alcohol or anyone's bed. She willingly accepted my offer of an extra session. At session 6 she was coping better, having deployed her two defences of 'battening the hatches down' and 'filling the day with activity'.

An examination success in which she had used all of her academic ability, successful confrontations with noisy library users and a neighbour, and the experience of being held like a child by a girlfriend accounted for her exuberant state the following week. She was more open to my image of her as someone who takes a strong motherly role and yet who wants to be mothered.

I arrived late for session 8. Understandably Mary was angry. She was, also, downcast and silent. Reluctantly and in tears she accused me of taking a sadistic delight in having broken her shell and exposed her dependency. 'Now you've got me squirming – I suppose it's part of the therapy.' I spoke of the need to integrate her valued independent and hated dependent self that she so wished to dispense with. She agreed that she was a 'person of extremes'. A contextual factor emerged: the end of the academic term and the impending loss of her life-structuring role as a student.

Easier ground had been reached in session 9. A key factor was a new man in her life, a gentle divorcee with whom she had in common the fact that he was a single parent. Mary was frightened by her attraction to him. She feared being swept away and getting hurt; it was safer to stay at one of her extremes: the extreme of isolation. I found myself urging her to go slowly; a justifiable caution, but also a reflection of my over-protective, almost possessive, feelings.

Looking back on these sessions, many new understandings occur to me. At the time, I attended to and emphasised Mary's way of being (practice point 4) in her reported world, i.e. in the world of current relationships external to the therapy room (practice points 2 and 4). Conversely my awareness of how caught up I was in a similar pattern within the room was at a preconscious level. The spotlight of my attention had not fully illuminated it; I did not see how my coming to know her was activating the pattern (practice point 8). I noticed to be sure that sometimes my psychological movements towards her were comforting and sometimes frightening, and deduced from this the conflict between her isolated, lonely self and her dependent hurtable self. I had confidence that the experience of better relationships would be the

corrective one which would reconcile her two extremes, and that this
new 'being' would primarily occur in the external world (practice
points 1, 4 and 5). My focus was outwards-directed towards, for example, exploring the conflictual relationship with her daughter. Here,
her difficulty in facing her resentment over the decision of her child of
5 to live with her former husband made sense when viewed against
Mary's imperative not to be possessive and controlling like her mother
(practice point 3). I did not attend to my strong engagement in the
repeated patterns of her story (practice point 6). I was inclined to
minimise the tension that flared up between us and, when I did address
it, my framework was historical.

The second phase

Her daughter visited during the vacation. This brought to the surface
resentful feelings that her life-space was being invaded. Life, once
more, seemed out of Mary's control. She had little money, which reduced her independence and hurt her pride. She had to provide for her
daughter, and the new man in her life was not proving as efficient as he
had first appeared. Memories from her childhood flooded up to be
discussed and pushed down again. She recalled two formative experiences: first, her mother stigmatising her for being partially deaf and,
secondly, feeling very much alone when she was admitted to hospital
at the age of 5.

I gradually became aware that certain of my comments were received as insensitive assaults. My intended message was of benevolent
interest in exploring her puzzling feelings, but the reception, for example, of anything I said about Terry, the well-regarded boyfriend of 2
years before who wanted Mary but not her daughter, was quite different. He understood her and made her sit down when she was upset
and say what she was really feeling. However, he also wanted his freedom to come and go as he pleased on the spur of the moment. I
questioned her portrayal of him as 'sensitive and concerned'. Was he
not a little selfish and had it not been insensitive to reply laconically to
her lonely letter 6 months before that he might see her in a couple of
years should his work bring him to her town? This communication was
rejected out of hand. My response was to rephrase it in ever more
tactful ways because it seemed that there was a truth to be faced or at
the very least considered. This modification also failed, and it was clear
to me that there was something that my way of practice was not taking
into account.

The next session began stickily. Mary was silent and could only think
negatively about herself. Her gloom was not lightened by my suggestion that she had been taught by someone to expect the worst. She
replied that she could remember nothing before the age of 10. At

length, her irritation surfaced. What was the point of her seeing me when her views were not accepted? I was telling her what to think and threatening to take away her precious memories of Terry. To myself, I thought that those who threaten another's idols do so at their peril. To Mary, I suggested that a central concern for her was not to be influenced. In a more accepting tone, she remembered at the age of 8 deciding to go her own way and not conform to her mother's wishes. I related this reaction against her mother's pressure to the inhibition that Mary felt about voicing her opposition when her daughter decided to move away. This seemed a likely direction and we wandered off down this path, temptingly smooth with room for two, and, perhaps, both a little relieved that we were on the easier ground of past relationships. With hindsight, I would have handled the situation differently and recognised that the jagged uncomfortable way was the main way, the road of central importance and change. I should have stayed with her feelings of outrage when I threatened to control her.

The pattern becomes clearer

Her lability of outlook and vulnerability to setbacks and her sensitivity to my presumed view of her were increasingly evident as each week went by. On return to college she regained her student role. The stream of study carried her on, but she hit against the rocks of isolation and being different. Some younger women cast her in the role of mother and protector, and confided to her their independent promiscuous lives. The tension in the room rose when Mary asked me what I thought of this promiscuity. I replied neutrally that, on the one hand, it could be a natural phase and, on the other, a driven need. I turned the conversation away from what I thought to what she thought of her promiscuous phase, her search for comfort.

Mary was irritated by the suggestion that she had a dependent self. She spoke of her difficult relationships with men. Some depended on her and she despised them for this (the unacceptable part of herself); these men suffocated her by wanting to control her (I wondered if this was a warning to me). Others were independent spirits and these she liked best; but with them, a time would come – often the time of ending – when she would want them to bend to her in some visible way. For Mary, for them to bend would signify her great value to them. But, of course, men chosen for their independent style continued in this way and Mary would be cast down into depression (practice points 2, 4 and 6). The dilemma of her inner extremes was played out in her intimate choices.

At our next meeting she was consumed with self-hate. I interpreted that she was only listening to the criticism from her mother that she had internalised. For a moment she could take in my words and feel unpersecuted enough to tell me how her mother was still saying that she was bad and still implying to her that life without a man was awful. Then, the moment was lost, and her anger flared. She accused me of pushing her back into the marriage slot in society. Feeling sinisterly transformed, I replied that this was her interpretation and that I did not recognise any such intent on my part. I made sense of what had happened by postulating that she had an inner murderous hate for her mother which she generally turned against herself and which surfaced when she felt others treated her in a hateful way. Mary was horrified. She had never thought that before and anyway such thoughts could not be entertained as her parents were 'poor old people'. We ended on a subdued note.

Paradox again entered into our next meaning. Mary felt sad and pessimistic. If she died no one would notice; no gap would be left. 'I would be sad', I truthfully replied. Mary grew angry. Out of this truthful, passionate exchange, layers of her being gave up their secrets. Being cared about provoked anger in her – anger at not having been loved by her parents as a child – and also a frightened longing for love now.

At our twentieth meeting, Mary was brighter. She had been thinking that as a child she had developed a false self (Laing, 1959) to please her parents and was only now bringing into view her inner self. Her parents relied upon her and assumed that they could continue so doing, which she resented. I wondered if she could not be more direct (practice point 6) and gradually undermine their illusion, but Mary was apprehensive that any confrontations would destroy them – they remained upset for months after any criticism. However, we both laughed when I joked that there might be poison in the cake that she was baking in preparation for a visit home.

The following week's session was hesitant, with Mary in low spirits and seeming to hang on to my words. My comment that her state might be a reaction to the sense of power to challenge her parents that she had toyed with the week before was not understood, and Mary started to talk in a small voice, crying and being critical of herself for not understanding my words. Again I felt that they were heard in a very different way than I intended, and interpreted the transference by linking her present way of talking with how she had spoken with her parents as a child (Malan, 1979). Childhood memories emerged, and the next week she had a fantasy which was both distressing and curiously relieving that she and her brother might be illegitimate and not really of the same blood as her parents.

Significant acts

In the middle and final thirds of therapy, Mary's relationships with men and friends offered many opportunities for significant acts of change (practice point 6). An early opportunity came with a move into a shared house with two fellow lodgers, one a man in his fifties and the other a single man of the same age as herself. The older man treated her like a young daughter and wanted to know the wheres and whats of her social life. The girlfriend of the younger man took a traditional female role and, much to Mary's annoyance, washed his shirts and spent hours in the kitchen cooking his meals. Mary felt trapped, her independence gone and her concept of her own femaleness threatened. She and I recognised that she was facing a recreation of some disliked aspects of her child-hood, and we discussed how she might redress the balance by setting limits to what she would answer and negotiating times for use of the kitchen. Our cooperative agreement was tinged with ambivalence on her part as she felt scared when I had noticed without her telling me how frightened she was. Were her defences so easily breached that others could see into her? As it turned out, *Kairos* (Kelman, 1969), the auspicious moment, had not arrived for successful significant acts and she moved back to her flat. She did, however, succeed in refusing to help her parents move house when they had already enlisted the aid of her brother and friends. A few weeks later she was to resist her mother babying her, and was able to hold her position despite her mother black-mailing her with tears; to her pleasant surprise, her father emerged from his background role to support her.

Two short-lived affairs brought all her fears to the surface. She went to a 'marvellous party' with one man, a recent divorcee, but was devas-tated when he would not meet her the next day. The hint of rejection was enough to make her literally run away in distress. The knowledge that he had a girlfriend and might adversely compare Mary sexually with her compounded the situation. She wanted to feel that he was committed to her. For me to suggest that caution might be prudent early in a relationship was to criticise her and take advantage of her vulnerability. This man drew back from Mary, saying that he could not cope with her sudden 'cutting-off' from him. (I found Mary's cutting-off from me at moments of understanding and concern equally disconcert-ing.) Another man seemed very promising but stunned her with the news that he was going to work in another town. It seemed clear to me that she was choosing men who were as apprehensive about commit-ment as herself; she endowed them with an idealised image, ignored the warning signs, and then was devastated when the end came. In contrast to the conditional love from her mother, she wanted to be prized as she was, but her longing for this and her fear when it began to happen confused her men and ultimately drove them away.

In the final 7 months, the same patterns recurred with an important new boyfriend, Stephen, but she was able to recognise the pattern, discuss with me what was going wrong and continue in the relationship while finding new solutions to old situations. How we passed from me being critic and attacker to collaborator and guide at moments of crisis is detailed in the next section. With Stephen, she learned to be more open and, for example, to risk alienating him by asking him to stay away when she wanted to be alone. She was no longer panicked into flight by the apparent breakdown in the relationship and was able to hold her ground and work through the innocent misunderstandings. Most significant of all was the fact that the relationship lasted, and when she finished therapy it was set to prosper.

Being known and the initiation of change

With Mary I walked a narrow, changing path. The way ahead was often black, and one or both of us were at fault for that. She revelled in the sun when it shone as it rarely did, but expected it not to last. At times of despair she railed against the inequality of therapy; it would be much easier if we met as friends, as equals; then, it would be less humiliating and frightening to show her hurt, needy self. One wrong word from me and I would be transformed into a repressive critic, a role that I found uncomfortable. My sensitivities had the beneficial effect of easily allow-ing me to understand her reactions, but worked against an early confrontation of the pattern when I saw how pained she was by disap-pointment (practice point 9). In terms of transference, I alternated between idealised friend and critical mother. Sullivan's (1970) concept of parataxic distortion captured how I felt; there would be dialogue between Mary and me – and then between Mary and a third, hateful person whom she regarded as being me. This sinister transformation happened again and again. I attempted to resist it by not accepting the new role or backing off and gently seeking to re-establish the collabora-tive relationship. However, the nicer I was, the more her underlying disappointment surfaced and the angrier and the more suspicious she became.

I came to see that these transformations were more than enactments of probable aspects of her relationship with her mother, but were manifestations of what went wrong with others and what was happen-ing between us. It was me as a person coming to know her as a person that was central. This knowing aroused all her fears and angry disap-pointments, which in turn called a halt to progress. Realising this al-lowed me to fight to be the person I am – not just the protective caring polarity that was encouraged by her idealisation and which she ul-timately needed, but to use the anger that I felt at being halted and transformed and to share with her the impact of her attacks.

Two examples may illustrate this change. At the mid-point of therapy her appointment was cancelled one week as I had a teaching commit-ment. She rang asking for an appointment that week. As the teaching event had been cancelled, I offered her through my secretary her usual time. Mary refused the offer. When we met the next week she was withdrawn, subdued and apologetic. She was reluctant to examine the recent happenings but eventually said how disappointed she had been; she had been refused, the refusal was absolute and her need had been urgent. Angered at being once more cast in an insensitive role, I pointed out that she had rights and that I would have made time if she had made clear the gravity of her need. Despite her disbelief, I insisted that this was true. Consequently, we both broke the repetitive, ultimately sterile pattern that we had formed. She neither withdrew feeling let down nor flared up like a child criticised, and I did not sit on the edge of my chair feeling that I had failed, had harmed and, now, must put right. A productive exchange followed in which the great significance to her of asking for extra was explored, as was the way in which she had invited disappointment by not being sufficiently direct. A few weeks later she was to test my 'good faith' by asking for and getting an extra session. Change had been initiated and the sequence of consolidation began.

It became progressively easier for us to recognise the pattern when it occurred between us, and to address it without resorting to defensive manoeuvres. There were still times when she felt controlled by me and experienced my drawing attention to the fear and anger she felt during holiday breaks from therapy as 'grinding her in the dirt', or reacted with resigned hostility when my perception of events differed from hers, but these grew less frequent. The last was another recreation of her childhood relationship with her parents, when it had been pointless for her to ask for what she wanted as it would have been refused, or she would be told that she did not mean what she had said. She became more direct and was able to determine the issues that she wished to address in a session. Her new decisiveness was reflected in similar actions outside therapy.

Some sessions later Mary felt sad and hurt when I did not understand something that she had said. She spoke of her resentment towards her parents and a fear that her anger, if expressed, would destroy them. She wanted to know what impact it had on me. I answered that it pinned me back into my chair, made me want to go away and left me feeling guilty over having been so clumsy or thoughtless. Then and now I think it was important to have answered directly. Answering as I did *and* at the right moment changed the relationship and freed us to explore together another area in our exchange, and opened up a fruitful examination of the same awkward moments with those in her external life to whom she drew close. It helped her gauge her impact and countered both her apprehension that she could destroy and, more importantly, that she was without influence.

Other guides

Within the narrow confines of the consulting room, it is all too easy for the therapist to over-value his or her centrality in the patient's life. It was thus salutary for me to learn in the second year of Mary's equally long-standing relationship with a fellow student, a widower in his sixties. In their friendship, she was daughter, friend and in fantasy perhaps lover. With him she found she could share her inner feelings, have her confidences respected and be accepted and be prized for what she offered (practice point 5). He was a guide to the high ground of good personal relationships. Her grief was great when he died of cancer. However, the good quality of that relationship paved the way for the sustained intimacy with her boyfriend Stephen.

The parting of the ways

The consideration of personal imagery and significant acts is an important component of my approach. I thus took great pleasure in the painting Mary brought me some weeks before termination. She had pictured herself as a tree with stunted roots and a brittle trunk. However, above, a few leaves sprouted which she linked to commencing therapy and then coloured branches, expanding, full of life and spreading off the sheet.

She went her way. She had graduated, she was looking for a post and hoped to share a home with Stephen. Six months later she sent me a Christmas card with her best wishes.

Emergent New Developments

The developments in my work as the result of this key case are extensions of my last two practice points: being known (practice point 8) and the personal history of the therapist (practice point 9). I continue to work practically with the interpersonal difficulties in the external world, but am much more aware of and comfortable in working in a personal way with these same difficulties when they occur between me and the patient. In this I emphasise more the personal and less the abstract historical aspects of the transference. My commitment to assisting with change in problematic relationship patterns in the patient's current life remains the same, but I now more fully appreciate the locus for change that exists within the therapy hour in the reality that patient and therapist create. Clearly this has historical antecedents on both sides, but it is in exploring the present experience of each other that much potential for change exists. I bring out my new learning in four further practice points, illustrated by work with a subsequent case.

Practice point 10: Moments for change occur at times of tension within the therapeutic relationship

As I know keenly from my work with Mary, there will be moments in therapy when the therapeutic alliance, the 'non-neurotic, rational, reasonable rapport which the patient has with his analyst and which enables him to work purposefully in the analytic situation' (Greenson and Wexler, 1969) is disrupted by tension; this is generally the product of negative feelings and inclines the patient or therapist or both to withdraw. Advancing into the jagged awkwardness of the tension is difficult but illuminating. It is in this moment that one potential for a corrective emotional experience (practice point 5) and initiation of change lies. Withdrawing is understandable but usually represents a lost opportunity. With Mary, it was only when I stopped pretending that we were at one that it was possible to examine how we had reached the brink of disaster – the breakdown of the relationship – and what the pattern of our interaction signified dynamically.

Practice point 11: Attend closely to the process of the sessions

Content and process are related elements in the sequence of the therapy sessions. Content is the subject matter which forms the readily apparent surface of the session. Process is the underlying, less than conscious, current that directs the content from moment to moment and session to session. The therapist who has a longitudinal perspective can decipher hidden important communications in the sequence of the content; he will be alert to messages about the therapy relationship conveyed in the form of stories told about external events or from alterations in emotional states or sudden changes in topic that are reactions to what has gone before. Subtle changes in emotional tone signal crucial interactions. As indicated (practice point 10), it is the awkward moments that are often the most illuminating; they arise out of assumptions (practice point 6) on either side somehow not being met. For the therapist, the feeling within the session is like running one's finger unexpectedly on a thorn or suddenly discovering that one has been cast in a drama quite different from the official play. My transformation with Mary from friend to repressive critic is one example; the alteration was triggered by minor failings to take the idealised role that she wished me to have with her.

Practice point 12: Consider how patient and therapist combine

How the therapist and patient combine in the exchange of therapy is a function of who they are as people. To the combination, the therapist contributes a certain role model learned in training, but of greater importance are his or her personal qualities and the engagement of interests and vulnerabilities by the patient's actions. The interface is formed by the interaction between the two psychological worlds of patient and therapist; both react out of their public and private selves, and *both* are involved in processes of appraising and confirming, valuing and rejecting, freeing and constraining. Understanding the different levels on which the therapist is engaged and having the confidence to use the reactions productively at the right time may convert negative aspects of the fit into positive ones.

With Mary, my protective tendency was enhanced by not wanting to see her hurt and not wanting to be the originator of that hurt. The relationship felt off-balance, and we were often close to failing. At the right time, that is, once sufficient trust had been built up through our repeated struggles, a rigorous appraisal of what was happening between us led to the more equal and mature relationship that Mary had desired.

Practice point 13: Be open to being moved by the patient

For many good and less than good reasons, the therapy relationship is fundamentally unequal in power (Heller, 1985). This may compound the patient's sense of powerlessness (practice point 1). Furthermore, the patient may doubt that he, his dilemmas and feelings have any impact on others, and if they have any impact, he may be unsure of its form. I have always conceptualised the therapeutic relationship as a dialectic where both may be changed; certainly both are moved by what passes between them. Now, I am more open in showing how I am moved.

In my second case, the way in which I showed my frailty illustrates this point and the other developments in practice.

A Second Case

I had been working for several months with a highly intelligent, schizoid young man. He had no friends and affected not to need any. Nevertheless an acquaintance becoming less friendly and thus psychologically moving away from him had precipitated an overdose. His father was an intensely critical, high-achieving man who wanted his children to achieve but who could not cope with their worries. As a child, the patient had learnt to defend by attack and felt more secure when, then and now, he penetrated the defences of others with rapier-like thusts. His problematic pattern of relationships and its likely origin were clear to me, but he was reluctant to accept my formulation. With me, he undermined my confidence by constantly denigrating the rationale and practice of therapy and manoeuvring me into the position of being the one to sort out his problems as if they had nothing to do with him. The more I strove to understand him, the more he denigrated my acts (practice point 11). In terms of process, being understood was for him the same as being vulnerable.

I began by interpreting the recreation of his family dynamics with myself in the role of dangerous father who must be rendered helpless, but to no avail. The interpretation was almost certainly historically correct, but it did not address what was happening in a way that permitted change. His thrusts continued; they penetrated my being and achieved their purpose. I was ready to give up. My omnipotent need led me, in my public self, to be calm and unperturbed, but this wore thin as the weeks went by (practice points 10 and 12). At length, I sued for peace. I said 'You can go on using your rapiers against me, and you are so good at it that you will defeat me and I will give up. I don't want that, but is that what you want?' (practice point 13). Initially he was outraged; I had no right to be upset and should be able to take anything. Later he became less attacking; he was even able to speak of his 'destitute' inner self. My unperturbed defence against being rendered helpless by his attacks had the effect of redoubling their ferocity (practice points 10 and 12). Revealing my frailty, while it appalled him, made me less dangerous and opened the way to productive work (practice point 13).

Implications for Other Therapists

It would be self-deceiving to suggest that the forward steps that I have taken have not been taken by other therapists. However, in the therapeutic landscape some are already on what seems to be a promising path and others could beneficially draw closer. It could also be that other guides have found equally good paths to the high ground of good relationships.

The implications of my learning are sixfold: (1) the advantages of synthesis; (2) the importance of the assumptive metaphor that we each have for our kind of therapy; (3) dialogue and authenticity as fundamental elements in the encounter of therapy; (4) the importance of adopting a structural approach to understanding the interactive product of the therapist and patient; (5) the value in promoting change of addressing the present rather than the historical aspects of the transference; and (6) a suggested model for identifying the relationship patterns that are difficult for the patient and which will be problematic in therapy.

Synthesis

Earlier I have stated my view that the intrapsychic and the interpersonal are indivisible (practice point 7). At least in their writings, many authors act as if this was not so and maintain that there is some primary good in concentrating on what seems to me to be one side of the same coin or, if you will, one end of a continuum. Kleinians consider all their patient's utterances as manifestations of transference, and turn away from considering the detail of the external world. Skinnerians deny the importance of inner experience and conceptualise individual actions as behaviours dictated by stimulus and reinforcement just as the puppet moves to pulls of the strings. I accept, of course, that in practice there is a gap between what therapists say they do and what they actually do; successful therapists are much more similar than different. However, these extreme positions are unreasonable. The twin focus of my approach is a strength. I consider equally the significant acts in the external world that a person makes and wishes to be able to make, and the inner world of meaning and dynamic origin. Adopting my position would circumvent much of the continuing sterile debate in which analysts criticise behaviourists for being superficial and behaviourists regard analysts as impractical fantasists. The way might then be open for each to learn from the other.

My work has a pragmatic contemporary emphasis on interpersonal problems and solutions. My two cases fit easily into my model, but then their interpersonal concerns are the concerns of our time. As Levinson (1972) has observed, patients change as the culture alters. The conversion hysterias that Freud saw are rare now. The existential *Angst* that dominated the 1960s and early 1970s has been superseded by concern with the quality of personal relationships.

Images of therapy

In this chapter I have proposed the images of therapy as a landscape which is explored and travelled through by patient and therapist; the journey is important for both. In a similar vein, Schafer (1983) describes the therapist as a seasoned, hardy guide to difficult places. Elsewhere (Aveline, 1980), I have explored the metaphor of the therapist as a good servant who puts his or her master's needs before his or her own and safeguards his or her best interest. Images are important. Hobson's (1985) concept of therapy as a conversation and Mair's (1977) of promoting dialogue with and among the patient's inner community of selves are implying a totally different relationship to that predicated on seeing the mind as a black box or supercomputer, or humankind as fallen angels. It behoves therapists to become aware of their assumptive metaphors and the roles that these prescribe. Freud (1938) saw the analyst as an archaeologist exploring into the patient's past and making constructions of what had existed before. This backward stance was in line with his view that one function of analysis was as a system of scientific enquiry; it paid relatively little attention to the present and the future.

Langs (1973) proposed the therapist as expert and healer and ca͟ tioned against stepping out of that role. He counsels the therapist t͟ maintain proper boundaries and be an effective, healthy, non-corrupt model for the patient; in this, he will guard himself against being seductive or hostile. I agree entirely with this intention: my highest ethical rule is 'Thou shalt not exploit the power relationship of therapy' – but I doubt the means. Overall, I find the image aseptic and cold, safe but unmoving.

Storr (1968) uses the image of an enigma.

> By keeping his own personality in the background and revealing as little of himself as possible, the analyst presents the patient with an enigma. The less the patient knows, the more will his picture of the analyst be coloured by his experience of people in the past; and the clearer will be the analyst's and the patient's perception of what has gone amiss with his previous relationships (p. 78).

I suggest that one can be enigmatic but not an enigma. Everything that one does, what one says, how one sits and the way in which the room is set out, reveals aspects of one's being which are the object of close, legitimate scrutiny by the patient. Indeed, as I have demonstrated in my examples, there is advantage in being, as Guntrip (1968) put it: 'a sufficiently real person to the patient to give him a chance of being a real person himself and not an assembly of defences, or a role, or a conforming mask, or a mass of unresolved tension' (p. 351). Guntrip predicated change on the patient meeting with personal reality in the therapist – a demanding task indeed!

Dialogue and authenticity

The line that I am developing is similar to that taken by Lomas (1981), although I cannot equal his openness as a therapist. Coming from psychoanalysis, he stresses in his work the value of ordinary responses to troubled people as well as the special knowledge unique to psychotherapy. Friendship is his paradigm for therapy rather than the application of scientific theory.

> The commonplace attitudes which are relevant to healing lie in the direction of warmth rather than coldness, trust rather than cynicism, closeness rather than distance, encouragement rather than discouragement, spontaneity rather than calculation.   Lomas, 1981, p. 6

Above all, he is humble and respectful; the same point is made by Greben (1981). Humanist existential writers, such as Rogers (1961), Buber (1958), May, Angel and Ellenberger (1958) and Yalom (1980), use the language of meeting and encounter. They point towards an

ig, an exploration of the 'in-between' and an experi-
her side. Jung saw therapy as a dialectical process
involved persons in which both were open to the other's
, both were engaged in enquiry and both contributed to the
experience (Fordham, 1979). In other words, Jung moved and
was moved by his patients. How much do other therapists allow this
vital movement?

A structural approach to the dynamics of the patient–therapist relationship

All therapists need to consider their contribution to the pattern that
emerges between them and their patient. The therapist is never a neutral figure, however much his theory encourages the belief in consistent scientific techniques (interventions and interpretations) with the
prime variability residing in the patient. Sullivan's (1953) term, the
'participant-observer', underlines this point. Long before, James (1950)
described the multiple social selves each of us has, and which are
differentially encouraged by certain people. Levinson (1972) argues
convincingly for a structural approach in which we can only understand what is happening by considering how the systems of patient,
therapist, family and society are mutually engaged. Each patient has a
private myth which transforms the therapist on contact and in which
the therapist is inevitably caught up. An authentic responsible recognition of what is happening may break the pattern and be a corrective
experience.

In my second case, there was a struggle for survival in which for a
while only one of us seemed likely to survive. I was cast in the role of
attacker, and needed for my sake to defend my existence. I did indeed
represent many of the values of the patient's father's generation. To
attempt to win through by exposing the patient's vulnerability was to
be an attacker. To abandon that role was to give him true power to
decide his own disclosures.

Transference and countertransference

With the concepts of transference and countertransference, Freud
made a most fundamental contribution to our thinking. In the examples
that I have cited, I recognise the importance of past perceived experience for present reactions and show how much my perception has
been shaped by the frame of transference. Indeed, paradoxically, these
two cases forcibly reminded me how much present patterns of interactions are facsimiles of past relationships with important others. The
traveller's tale of the psychoanalyst made more sense to me than ever
before. However, only when, in a very ordinary way, the current reality

was addressed, rather than the historical antecedents, did the pattern change. History provides us with understanding, but insight is not synonymous with personal change.

Transference is a useful way of ordering what happens, but may be seized upon by the therapist to distance him- or herself from the awkward moments I have described. In the same way, the person as a person may be lost in the higher order constructs of psychopathology. For the therapist and patient alike, the awkwardness of being known may be attributed to there-and-then relationships with parents that are safely past, rather than to something that is happening now. In contrast, addressing the emotional reality of the here-and-now is therapeutically influential. Further ways of advancing towards the important goal of a transference-free relationship in therapy can be achieved by supporting the patient's observing ego through accepting correct perceptions, especially of therapist deficiencies, openly admitting efforts, avoiding arrogance and explaining the rationale of procedures (Greenson and Wexler, 1969).

Identifying likely problematic relationship patterns within therapy

Many combinations of therapist and patient fail. Negative patterns develop and are not resolved. Attempts to ignore what is happening, or merely to interpret the historical antecedents, frequently – as in my two cases – fail to resolve the impending impasse. But, it is often difficult to perceive the pattern in which one is or will be caught up.

In an exciting innovation, Strupp and Binder (1984) have found a way of describing in narrative form what characteristically happens between a patient and others. These interpersonal transactions are historically significant and sources of current difficulty. Using the patient's words, the therapist constructs that person's characteristic interpersonal narrative. The narrative begins with interpersonal acts committed by the patient. In the second place the expectations that that person has about the reactions of others to him or her are documented. Third, the consequently observed actions of others are noted, as is how the patient then acts towards himself. Such a model would have been very useful to me in my work with Mary. Its atheoretical approach may prove very useful to therapists of many persuasions, and especially to those interested in the vicissitudes of interpersonal processes.

When the relationship is in trouble, directly addressing the problematic feelings that the patient has about the therapist can be helpful (Foreman and Marmar, 1985). This may be enough to join the paths once more. What has to be recognised is the nature of the psychotherapy undertaking. In this endeavour, in the final analysis, patient and therapist are ordinary mortals. The patient is engaged in a process of being known, and will defend against this by enlisting the therapist in the service of his private myths. Working with the reality that exists between them is a way of change.

References

ADLER, A. (1924). *The Practice and Theory of Individual Psychology*. Transl. P. Radin. London: Kegan Paul.

ALEXANDER, F. and FRENCH, T. (1946). *Psychoanalytic Therapy: Principles and Applications*. New York: Ronald Press.

AVELINE, M.O. (1980). The therapist as the servant of the patient. Paper read to Psychotherapy Societies in Adelaide and Sydney.

AVELINE, M.O. (1984). Books reconsidered: persuasion and healing: J.D. Frank. *British Journal of Psychiatry*, **145**, 207–211.

AVELINE, M.O. (1986) The corrective emotional experience in psychotherapy: a fundamental unifying concept. Paper presented at the Annual Conference of the Society for Psychotherapy Research, Wellesley College, Massachusetts, June 1986.

AVELINE, M.O. and SMITH, J. (1986). Psychotherapy pre-assessment interview questionnaires: form, content and therapeutic impact. Paper presented at the Annual Conference of the Society for Psychotherapy Research, Wellesley, Massachusetts, June 1986.

BINSWANGER, L. (1956). Existential analysis and psychotherapy in F. Fromm-Reichmann and J. Moreno (Eds), *Progress in Psychotherapy*. New York: Grune & Stratton.

BUBER, M. (1958). *I and Thou*, 2nd edn. New York: Charles Scribner.

FORDHAM, M. (1979). Analytic psychology and counter-transference. In L. Epstein and A.H. Feiner (Eds), *Counter-transference: The Therapist's Contribution to the Therapeutic Situation*. New York: Jason Aronson.

FOREMAN, S.A. and MARMAR, C.R. (1985). Therapists' actions that address initially poor therapeutic alliances in psychotherapy. *American Journal of Psychiatry* **142**, 922–926.

FRANK, J.D. (1973). *Persuasion and Healing*, 2nd edn. New York: Schocken Books.

FREUD, S. (1938). Construction in analysis. *International Journal of Psychoanalysis* **19**, 377–387.

GREBEN, S.E. (1981). The essence of psychotherapy. *British Journal of Psychiatry* **138**, 449–455.

GREENSON, R.R. and WEXLER, M. (1969). The non-transference relationship in the psychoanalytic situation. *International Journal of Psychoanalysis* **50**, 27–39.

GUNTRIP, H. (1968). *Schizoid Phenomena, Object Relations and Self*. London: Hogarth Press.

HEIDEGGER, M. (1962). *Being and Time*. Transl. J. Macquarre and E. Robinson. New York: Harper & Row.

HELLER, D. (1985). *Power in Psychotherapeutic Practice*. New York: Human Sciences Press.

HOBSON, R.F. (1985). *Forms of Feeling: The Heart of Psychotherapy*. London: Tavistock.

HORNEY, K. (1945). *Our Inner Conflicts*. New York: W.W. Norton.

JAMES, W. (1950). *The Principles of Psychology*, vol. 1. New York: Dover Publications.

KELMAN, H. (1969). Kairos: the auspicious moment. *American Journal of Psychoanalysis* **29**, 59–83.

LAING, R.D. (1959). *The Divided Self*. London: Tavistock.

LANGS, R. (1973). *The Technique of Psychoanalytic Psychotherapy*, vol. I. New York: Jason Aronson.

LEVINSON, E.A. (1972). *The Fallacy of Understanding*. New York: Basic Books.

LOMAS, P. (1981). *The Case for a Personal Psychotherapy*. Oxford: Oxford University Press.

MAIR, M. (1977). The community of self. In D. Bannister (Ed.), *New Perspectives in Personal Construct Theory*. New York: Academic Press.

MALAN, D.H. (1979). *Individual Psychotherapy and the Science of Psychodynamics*. London: Butterworths.

MAY, R., ANGEL, E. and ELLENBERGER, H.E. (1958). *Existence: A New Dimension in Psychiatry and Psychology*. New York: Basic Books.

ROGERS, C.R. (1961). *On Becoming a Person*. London: Constable.

SCHAFER, R. (1983). *The Analytic Attitude*. London: Hogarth Press.

STORR, A. (1968). The concept of care. In C. Rycroft (Ed.), *Psychoanalysis Observed*. London: Pelican Books.

STRUPP, H.H. and BINDER, J.L. (1984). *Psychotherapy in a New Key*. New York: Basic Books.

SULLIVAN, H.S. (1953). *The Interpersonal Theory of Psychiatry*. New York: Basic Books.

SULLIVAN, H.S. (1970). *The Psychiatric Interview*. New York: W.W. Norton.

YALOM, I.D. (1980). *Existential Psychotherapy*. New York: Basic Books.

Chapter 3
The Provision of Illusion in Psychotherapy

An important element in successful psychotherapy is the provision of illusion. By illusion, I mean the misinterpretation of events by the therapist for the purpose of furthering therapy. Why this should be necessary will, I hope, become clear as I develop this proposition.

The departure point for this paper is one of those ambivalent and cruel cartoons about psychiatrists, psychoanalysts and their patients that regularly appear in the *New Yorker* and *Punch* magazine. The cartoon showed a patient, a little man, dishevelled, anxious and clearly inept, in the office of a psychiatrist. In contrast, the psychiatrist is large and impressive; he sits on a raised chair behind a vast desk. He is surrounded by the framed certificates of his competence. The patient asks 'Doctor, I keep on getting these feelings of inferiority. Why is this?'. The doctor replies, 'Because you *are* inferior'.

The doctor stakes out his claim to superiority by displaying the trappings of success, but the cartoon points to one of the unspoken and unspeakable dilemmas in psychotherapy. The dilemma is not that some people are inferior but that many of the people whom we attempt to help are in some way unlikeable, unpleasant and inept and, as I shall argue, encourage others to treat them as such. They may be, and often are, that way for very good reasons of genetic disadvantage or harsh and inhibiting rearing, reasons which once we know them stir our sympathy and summon our caring.

But this does not alter the fact that in circumstances other than a therapeutic relationship, we might well not seek them out as friends or soulmates. It does not alter the fact that each person is to a significant degree the architect of his or her own fate, caught in the grip of the compulsion to repeat his or her history which is so well described in

From M.O. Aveline (1989) The provision of illusion in psychotherapy. *Midland Journal of Psychotherapy* 1, 9–16, with permission.

psychoanalysis. The alienation and the isolation that they experience is largely engendered by themselves; their dissatisfaction results from their way of handling the ordinary encounters of living; the withdrawal or disapproval of others is a normal, even sensible, response to this.

The converse is equally familiar. The patient is decidedly more able, attractive or successful than ourselves, and we have to struggle to contain our envy or curb our narcissistic pleasure in having the company of that person.

And yet, our patients are seeking help to change their maladaptive strategies for coping, strategies which, even if recognised by them as not being in their best interest, cannot easily be dismissed or new ones commanded into being. Within therapy, they will manifest these archaic ways and unless something special happens, the old result will follow. That something special is the provision of illusion. The therapist suspends some of the normal rules of interaction; he does not reply in kind to the negative interpretations that are being placed upon his behaviour and reactions, does not take up the invitations, seductive or otherwise, that are being extended. Instead he recognises these behaviours for what they are and relates both to the person as he or she is, *and* to a hidden person in the patient, a more competent, likeable and cooperative self, a self that has partially emerged or which the therapist believes to be there (see Chapter 7). At the least, this manoeuvre provides an interregnum which enables therapy to proceed till the new self is established. At a more significant level, it may be a vital element in achieving change.

Maintaining the illusion is not easy. Factors first within the patient and secondly within the therapist destroy it. Fortunate is the therapist who is fired by optimism about his fellow man or, as Antony Storr (1979) puts it, has an 'irrational prejudice in favour of . . . the damaged, the despised, the insulted and the injured'. Faced with this problem, Jung (1932) advocated an attitude of 'unprejudiced objectivity', the cultivation of a 'deep respect for the facts, for the man who suffers from them, and for the riddle of such a man's life'.

As therapists, we strive to find likeable aspects in our patients to offset the less likeable aspects. We maintain our therapeutic stance by limiting the time we spend with them and turn for our support to supervision, conceptual theory – particularly conceptual theory that locates responsibility for current action outside the individual, often in the distant past of the patient – and, rarely but fruitfully, to role theory.

Factors in the Patient

In the 1930s, Franz Alexander in Chicago put forward the innovative concept of the 'corrective emotional experience' (Alexander and

French, 1946). By this, he meant the patient living through an experience in the here-and-now of therapy (or in his external life), similar in form to an earlier disappointing experience but this time with a new, more satisfying outcome, which would then correct the earlier maladaptive learning. For this to happen, the patient must first relive or enact historically meaningful patterns with the therapist, and second, be guided to new resolutions (Aveline, 1986).

So far so good. The therapist is instructed to maintain what Freud (1912) called an 'evenly suspended attention', to show neutrality, understanding, respect and decency, and to avoid sitting in judgement. In practice, as we all know, this is not easy. We mess it up in two ways: we either get caught up in the process of what is happening – the phenomenon of negative fit – or, defensively, prevent it happening at all.

Negative fit was first described by Luborsky and his colleagues (Luborsky et al., 1971; L. Luborsky and B. Singer, 1974, unpublished manuscript). In studying the process of therapy conducted by experienced therapists, they noticed that in a significant number of cases the therapist responded to the patient in ways that fitted the patients' negative expectations. Their behaviour confirmed the negative preconceptions, the inhibiting fears and malexpectations of the patient. Though there were many varieties of response, two types of negative fit predominated. Either the therapist confirmed the patient's fear of rejection by being critical, disapproving, condescending, ungiving, detached or super-neutral – that is, they showed an active lack of acceptance or a definite attitude of disinterest. Or they confirmed the patients' expectation of being made weak and dependent by being too directive, domineering and controlling.

Therapists have difficulty in perceiving that negative fit is occurring, and even greater difficulty in modifying the process. There is, however, evidence to suggest that meaningful and effective therapy cannot commence until a degree of negative fit is established. The skill in therapy lies in the ability to recognise what is happening, and then use what is happening constructively.

Hans Strupp (1977) has argued along these lines. He postulates that the 'unique contribution' of the therapist is 'in the skilful management of the interpersonal relationship for the purpose of achieving therapeutic change'. In his view, many of the techniques of traditional analytic therapy refer to ways of handling strategies and manoeuvres that the patient initiates and which are to be avoided. The therapist is taught, for example, to avoid being overprotective, to avoid being drawn into power struggles, to avoid participating in the neurotic games of the patient, games which are the essence of his illness. He encourages the patient to behave, in Haley's (1963) word, symptomatically, and then he frustrates these games by non-participation. Ultimately he poses to the patient a choice of retaining his maladaptive patterns with the consequence of losing the therapeutic relationship, or relinquishing his patterns as being anachronistic, unrealistic and based upon a gross misperception of the current situation, with the immediate benefit of retaining the relationship with his therapist, a relationship which by now he values. Which way the choice goes may well depend upon the quality of the real relationship between the two of them (Greben, 1984).

Factors within the Therapist

The patient exerts a powerful influence on the therapist. Heller, Myers and Kline (1963) in a role-play study demonstrated that interviewers responded with friendliness to friendly clients, with hostility to hostile clients, with passivity to dominant clients, and with activity and dominance to passive clients.

How therapists react to the patient significantly determines diagnosis and treatment. Strupp (1958) showed a film of an initial interview to 134 therapists and asked them at various important moments to record the responses that they would have made. The results were correlated with a post-interview questionnaire, prognosis, and with information about the therapists' training. Those therapists who disliked the patient tended to describe them in pejorative terms and with a poor prognosis. The treatment that they advised was stricter and briefer. They anticipated more problems. In contrast, therapists who liked the patient were more positive in all their comments.

There is no doubt in my mind that this finding is not unique to psychotherapists. I feel confident that a study of psychiatrists using organic or other conceptual frameworks would have illustrated a similar expression of responses and prejudices.

Unresolved conflicts within the therapist are a major limiting factor. This was shown in Bandura, Lipsher and Miller's classic (1960) paper on approach-avoidance reaction to the expression of hostility by patients. They studied the reaction of 12 postgraduate psychology students who were undertaking psychotherapy. Therapists who were able directly to express their own hostility in ordinary life, tolerated their patients' hostility well and did not inhibit its expression, but therapists who had a high need for approval avoided their patients' hostility, and often after a while these patients decreased the amount of hostility they expressed. Here, what happened resulted from a complex interplay between the behaviour of the patient and the countertransference of the therapist.

Similarly, a study by Cutler (1958) indicated that therapists were less effective in exploring areas that were problems for them as well as the patient, and were less accurate in telling their supervisors about it!

An interesting finding in Strupp's (1958) study that lends some support to the contention that training is worthwhile, was in the difference between therapists who had a personal analysis and those who had not. The analysed therapists were no less likely to dislike the patient than their unanalysed colleagues, but did show a greater capacity to conceal that dislike and to convey warmth and empathy.

Having described some of the implications of countertransference reactions, I now present the effect of more general perceptions and expectations that may be held by the therapist, perceptions which are not specifically triggered by the uniqueness of that patient but which are assumptions that colour the therapist's perception and usually limit his vision of what is possible for that patient.

In the cartoon that I described, the dice were loaded in favour of the psychiatrist. His sense of superiority was reinforced by the trappings of his success. There was no opportunity for the patient to demonstrate his successes, and indeed the very focusing on problems may, unless the psychiatrist or psychotherapist takes care to prevent it, preclude the discovery of personal abilities and assets that the patient has. In our work, we only see the wounded and their wounds.

The point that I am making is well illustrated in the phenomenon of institutionalisation among those who reside for a long time in mental hospitals. In 1959 Russell Barton published his account of institutional neurosis. He described a syndrome of gross apathy, inertia and self-neglect; the patients' horizons were limited and their capacity for decision-making atrophied. Barton asserted that this state was not the inevitable consequence of the schizophrenic process, but was largely a function of the attitudes of the staff and the way in which the institution was run. To a significant extent, his assertion has been confirmed. In 1970, John Wing and George Brown published the summation of their comparative study of the social treatment of schizophrenia in three English mental hospitals. In the original investigation, the level of social adjustment and the progression towards social adjustment over a 5-year period varied by as much as 50% between the hospitals. Nottingham pride compels me to relate that the hospital that did best was my own, Mapperley Hospital.

Basically, the factors that contributed to the better outcome were twofold: first, the attitude of seeing the patient as a person with rights and individuality, and secondly the practice of allowing, even insisting on, the exercise of an appropriate degree of personal responsibility and individual choice. These factors undercut the self-fulfilling negative prophecy from which these patients would otherwise have suffered and, in so doing, minimised the negative features of the chronic schizophrenia syndrome.

Role Theory

Role theory makes a useful contribution to understanding the nature of self-fulfilling prophecy. The sociologist, Irving Goffman, has long been interested in the interaction patterns that operate within asylums and other total institutions. One of his monographs (Goffman, 1959) concerns role, role embracement and role detachment. Technically, being in role means complying with all the normative expectations of others and, by definition, excluding anything from the presentation of self that is truly one's own, unless that complies with the demands of other people. We are all subject to role expectations. Some years ago, I lay in bed with 'flu and decided for the first time in my life to grow a beard. Once it was established, people said approvingly to me 'Now you are a proper psychotherapist!'.

In role embracement, the individual fuses with his role does not question it, and that role becomes his identity through and through. The institutionalised schizophrenic and the criminal serving a life sentence enter this role state. The personality labelled as psychopathic, hysterical or inadequate is held in the grip of powerful negative expectations which compound his natural tendency to embrace his role as a deviant or as a loser.

An intermediate state is that of role adoption: the individual temporarily takes on a role that is not truthful but which is socially adaptive. In fairgrounds, there are people called shrills: the busker drums up custom for his sideshow by singing its praises; the shrills rush forward and buy tickets. Onlookers are drawn by this show and buy tickets. What they do not know is that afterwards the shrills have their money refunded. Another example, nearer home, is at parties when, usually, the wife listens attentively, freshly and with amusement to her husband's jokes which she has surely heard a thousand times before. The pay-off is in easing the social situation and getting the party going.

In certain settings, particularly where the power of the individual is limited, role embracement can have damaging consequences. An important defence against it is role detachment. A person indicates subtly that the role he is performing is not truly him. He distances himself from this role. A subordinate taking instructions may indicate his independence by sullenness, muttering, irony, joking and sarcasm. The husband doing the washing up may perform it clumsily or ironically. In *One Flew over the Cuckoo's Nest*, the staff needed to take no notice of Chief Bromden for he was deaf and mute, when really he was neither.

Establishing role distance can be vital in coping with constraining situations. Caroline Moorehead in 1980 published a fascinating book about kidnapping. Geoffrey Jackson, the British Ambassador to Uruguay, was held prisoner by the Tupamaros for a year. He survived through a conscious decision to maintain his role distance. He refused to answer to 'Numero Uno' but would reply to 'Signor' or 'Jackson'. He would not join in any derogatory conversations about the Queen. Even though his food ration was barely sufficient, he put aside a portion each day so as to preserve his independence and as a test of his autonomous will. In contrast, Alberto Mori, the Italian Prime Minister, succumbed to the role pressure of his captors, the Red Brigade. He embraced the frightened helplessness that they intended; in his dependence upon them, he wrote pleading letters to the press and colleagues, letters of the sort he knew his own government had rejected in the past. Sadly, he was murdered in the end.

To return to the patient in the cartoon, his state in life was partly determined by the person he was and partly by the role expectations of others. He may have offered an inferior self, but for him to embrace the role definition of the psychiatrist as being inferior would be disastrous.

Conclusion

In the drama of therapy, both patient and therapist need to consider the pattern that they are forming together. Both may need to take action that will foster the intended good end of therapy.

For the patient, self-preservation is important. I thoroughly support Strupp, Hadley and Gomes-Schwartz's (1977) proposal of what amounts to a patients' charter. Two of their five points are relevant to this discussion. First, they advise the patient to be selective in his choice of therapist: to choose a therapist whose approach is consonant with the patient's own goals, resources and values. They say 'Make sure the therapist impresses you as a decent human being whom you can trust'. Secondly, the experience of intense, negative emotions during therapy, which discussion does not reduce, should prompt the patient to question the value of this therapy and consider changing to another therapist.

In the training of the psychotherapist, careful attention needs to be paid to the phenomenon of negative fit, problematic countertransference and negative role expectations. With regard to the last, it would be facile to suggest that change automatically follows when the therapist makes the mental leap to relate, not only to the patient's offered problematic self, but also to the hidden, more able self. Equally, the offered reality of the patient must be addressed: its form, meaning, historical origins and present consequences; to do otherwise would be to avoid grappling with the uncomfortable reality that constitutes the patient's problem. The therapist does not put on blinkers but holds to a greater vision, often in the face of many invitations to adopt a limited one. This greater vision maintains the therapeutic frame when it is threatened by discomforting interactions and, as I have argued, is an essential ingredient in the process of successful psychotherapy.

At all times, life presents many opportunities for a person to depart from the path that he or she has hitherto trod. The cross-roads are there for those who can see them and who have the courage to take the new direction. It is usually a major step of reorientation for the patient to build within himself a sufficient confidence in his ability to make changes in his life. To believe in himself, he needs to be believed in by a trusted companion, his therapist. At the same time, it is important for the therapist not to be over-optimistic about the extent of the change that is possible, or the rapidity with which it can be achieved, lest this view becomes a burdensome expectation for the patient and a further source of failure.

Thus, our sensitive, well-trained psychotherapist is fully aware of the dangers of reinforcing the patient's sense of inadequacy through the non-verbal medium of his surroundings, and through unspoken negative role expectations which command a harmful role embracement. He adopts a democratic style, comes out from behind his desk and sits alongside the patient. Face to face, they work together on the problems. A crucial element in their work is identifying the role that the patient has embraced and encouraging him to distance himself from it: to change, for example 'This is the way life has always been for me and I know it is going to go on in the same way' to 'This has been my experience but I don't have to have it as my future'. The therapeutic message is at one level conveyed through open conversation, but more insistently by the attitude of the therapist, which implies that a new role, different from the present one, is feasible for the patient and attainable by him. To return to the theme of my title, what is illusion today is reality tomorrow.

In conclusion, I quote from Goethe – at least, the attribution when I encountered the quotation was to Goethe, but I have never been able to find, and would dearly like to find, the source: 'If you relate to a man as he is, you make him worse. If you relate to him as he could be, you set him free to be that person.'

References

ALEXANDER, R. and FRENCH, T. (1946). *Psychoanalytic Therapy: Principles and Applications*. New York: Ronald Press.

AVELINE, M.O. (1986) The corrective emotional experience, a fundamental unifying concept in psychotherapy. Paper presented at the Annual Conference of the Society for Psychotherapy Research, Wellesley College, Massachusetts, June 1986.

BANDURA, A., LIPSHER, D.M. and MILLER, P.E. (1960). Psychotherapists approach-avoidance reactions to patients expression of hostility. *Journal of Consulting Psychology* 24, 1–8.

BARTON, R. (1959). *Institutional Neurosis*. Bristol: John Wright & Sons.

CUTLER, R.L. (1985). Counter-transference effects in psychotherapy. *Journal of Consulting Psychology* **22**, 349–356.

FREUD, S. (1912). *Recommendations to Physicians Practising Pychoanalysis,* vol. 12. London: Hogarth Press.

GREBEN, S.E. (1984). *Love's Labour.* New York: Shoken Books.

HALEY, J. (1963). *Strategies of Psychotherapy.* New York: Grune & Stratton.

HELLER, K., MYERS, R.A. and KLINE, L.V. (1963). Interview behavour as a function of standardised client roles. *Journal of Consulting Psychology* **27**, 117–122.

JUNG, C.G. (1932). *Psychotherapists or the Clergy in Psychology and Religion. Collected Works,* Vol. 11. London: Routledge & Kegan Paul.

LUBORSKY, L., CHANDLER, M., AUERBACH, A., COHEN, J. and BACHRACH, H.M. (1971). Factors influencing the outcome of psychotherapy. A review of quantitative research. *Psychological Bulletin* **75**, 145–185.

MOOREHEAD, C. (1980). *Fortune's Hostages: Kidnapping in the World Today.* London: Hamish Hamilton.

STORR, A. (1979). *The Art of Psychotherapy.* London: Secker & Warburg, Heinemann.

STRUPP, H.H. (1958). The psychotherapist's contribution to the treatment process. *Behavioural Science* **3**, 34–67.

STRUPP, H.H. (1977). A reformulation of the dynamics of the therapist's contribution. In: A.S. Gurman and A.M. Razin (Eds) *Effective Psychotherapy*, Chapter 1. Oxford: Pergamon Press.

STRUPP, H.H., HADLEY, S.W. and GOMES-SCHWARTZ, B. (1977). *Psychotherapy for Better or Worse. The Problem and Negative Effects.* New York: Jason, Aronson.

WING, J.K. and BROWN, G.W. (1970). *Institutionalism and Schizophrenia.* London: Cambridge University Press.

Chapter 4
Parameters of Danger: Interactive Elements in the Therapy Dyad

Introduction

For the purpose of this paper, a dangerous interaction between therapist and patient is taken to be one that completes the self-destructive, personally characteristic relationship pattern of the patient to a destructive degree. Typical destructive results are when the patient ends up feeling (1) rejected, (2) weak or (3) having had his or her boundaries inappropriately breached, sexually or emotionally. As I see it, the purpose of therapy is to help the patient write for him- or herself new, less destructive ends to old, sad stories (see Chapter 5). However, in the interactive dyad of therapist and patient, this good end does not always happen. Two questions arise which are important for all therapists, but especially for the beginning therapist and the supervisor:

1. Can the problematic, recurrent interpersonal patterns be identified for the patient and therapist alike?
2. Can potentially dangerous interactive patterns between a particular patient and a particular therapist be identified in advance and productively worked with?

Some partial answers to these questions are presented and the importance asserted of considering the combinations of therapists and patients that we, as supervisors and directors of training, bring together. The paper is in five sections. The first deals with our divided but nearly equal responsibility to patient and trainee. Then, an interpersonal perspective is outlined, as this provides a theoretical stance for understanding interactions; this is followed by a section on the concept of negative fit. The next focus is my context as a psychotherapy trainer within the National

This is from a presentation at the First Tavistock Clinic Symposium on Supervision, 4 August 1987.

Health Service in Nottingham, and the steps that we take to prepare beginning therapists for their first case. Finally, I present an outline of a therapy dyad where the interaction was damaging.

A Divided, Nearly Equal Responsibility

As clinicians, we have a primary responsibility to the patient to ensure that the person receives the best possible care. As trainers, we have a nearly equal responsibility to the beginning therapist to launch the trainee successfully on the path that passes through the four stages described by Hess (1986), from inception to skills development to consolidation and, finally, to mutuality. The first stage, which is the theme of this conference, is a time of much anxiety, insecurity and dependence on the supervisor, in which the therapist feels a mixture of ambivalent excitement and dread on seeing the first patient (Blount and Glenwick, 1982). The underlying issue is one of adequacy versus inadequacy, and is painfully pointed up by my case example. Part of our responsibility as trainers in trying to launch the trainee successfully is to combine that trainee with a patient who presents an appropriate level of difficulty, and where the result may be a mutually good experience.

We know that many therapists go wrong, but often we locate the problem in the patient, or in the therapist for not applying the technique properly. My argument is that there is all too frequently a mismatch between the two which is not recognised, and then the best course is, often, to change the pair. This uncoupling is rarely done, and probably should be done much more frequently. Even better, if one had great clarity of foresight, would be not to unite the two in the first place.

Strupp, Hadley and Gomes-Schwartz (1977), in their fascinating survey of factors identified by experienced therapists as contributing to negative effects in psychotherapy, identified two broad groups, one concerning the patient and the other concerning the therapist. In the patient, inaccurate assessment may lead to the therapy probing too deep or, conversely, cheating the patient by assuming a greater degree of fragility than actually exists. Ego strength and motivation may be lower than assessed, and there may be masochistic aspects of the patient which are summoned up by the process of therapy and acted out. The last needs to be seen in conjunction with a selection of the identified therapist factors. These include personality traits which are activated in the therapy dyad – voyeurism, sadomasochism, excessive unconscious hostility, seductiveness, pessimism and coldness. Negative effects may stem from technical rigidity, being overly intense and failing to maintain professional distance.

Happily, most therapists are well disposed towards their patients, although they often idealise their role and underestimate the difficulties in maintaining an affirmative relationship. The word *affirmative* is important, as it points to an essential contribution that the therapist can, and in my view has, to make (Schafer, 1983). When negative effects do occur, we would do well to consider the dyad as a whole.

An Interpersonal Perspective

Sullivan was the most thoroughgoing proponent of the theory that what happens between people is the product of their interactions and not just the result of fixed personality traits that operate across all situations. Of course, any one person demonstrates considerable consistency in his or her interactions, but we are speaking of complexity within consistency.

I share Sullivan's concern with personality. Sullivan considered personality to be the reflection of significant past relationships, and indeed stated that the patient's personality is the history. In the context of this paper, history is also what happens recurrently between patient and therapist. 'If you are to correctly understand your patient's problems', Sullivan declared, 'you must understand him in the major characteristics of his dealing with people' (Sullivan, 1970, p. 13).

In this framework, anxiety signals a threat to self-esteem and inner security, and is dealt with by selective distortion and inattention. The origins of the difficulties are indicated by parataxic distortion, which is a wider concept than transference and is close to Racker's (1968) concept of transferential predisposition. Thus the therapist is treated as if he were a person from the patient's past, but who may or may not have been the most important person from that past; the distortion depends upon who the other (in this case the therapist) is, and the context in which they meet.

This perspective leads to a distinctive style of therapy in which the task of the therapist is to stimulate curiosity in the patient about himself (just as the supervisor stimulates the same curiosity in the trainee), and to help the patient clarify his pattern of interaction, the distortions that exist in the patient's perceptions and the purposes these serve. The therapist joins with the patient in undertaking a detailed, active collaborative enquiry, in which the major source of the data is what transpires between the two (Cooper and Witenberg, 1984). Naturally, the therapy is conducted within a clear ethical frame.

One further aspect of Sullivanian theory fleshes out this interpersonal perspective. In his theorem of the reciprocal emotion, he pointed to the way in which within relationships the needs of both parties may be gratified or aggravated and, accordingly, the relationship may flourish or die. In therapy, the therapist is both observer and participant.

Research evidence, published as long ago as the early 1960s, has provided confirmatory evidence of the applicability of this theorem (Heller, Myers and Kline, 1963; Bohn, 1965). Therapists were observed to respond with friendliners to friendly clients, with hostility to hostile clients, with passivity to dominant clients, and with activity and dominance to passive clients.

In my own work, I know well how interactions with different people bring out different aspects of my being, often to my discomfort but always to my interest. In one recent case (see Chapter 2) a young man had been brought up in a house where family members used words like rapiers to attack and disable each other. There was no sense of the family being a welcoming, comforting place, and my patient carried this attitude into his adult life, where he was scornful of others and denied the existence of any dependent needs in himself. However, he was depressed and disturbed by feelings of loneliness that occasionally surfaced. He had a great need to protect himself from feeling and from being in a weak position, by the defence of taking control and undermining others. This pattern was repeated with me. From the outset, I felt on the defensive and found myself having to justify my position. My own need to be in control was threatened and I found myself reacting in an ever more reasonable, unperturbed manner, which only served to increase the ferocity of his attacks. These attacks penetrated my being to the point where I had to sue for peace. It was at this moment of breakdown in the relationship that we were able to escape from the escalating cycle of attack and my trying to appear to be unaffected, through the act of admitting my frailty. Initially he was appalled by this revelation, but then settled to some productive work as I became a less dangerous person in his eyes. In another case, a sadistic part of myself was engaged by the deferential, obedient manner of a female patient. Her childhood experience had been of a fierce, critical mother who was ready to blame her and favour her peers. My patient's coping pattern was one of external appeasement and inward, inhibited rage with the control that her mother and others in a similar psychological position exercised over her. With me, as the end of the session approached, I only had to look at the clock for her to leap to her feet in mid-sentence and apologetically leave the room. It was all too tempting to complete her pattern by taking the role of attacking mother. It is therapeutic to stop and look with her at what was happening, and to relate this to the way in which she, in her contemporary life, encouraged older women to complete her pattern by being hateful controllers.

In this section, the final point of theory to be raised is the corrective emotional experience as described by Alexander and French (1946). Here, the essence of the concept is a lived experience of a different end to a habitual, sad story (Aveline, unpublished data). In my first example, the corrective experience in the therapy was of my frailty and my wish to continue in coming to know him despite my extreme discomfort. In the second example, her being able to challenge me without being counterattacked was one important element in the process of change. The question then arises: if we can identify what would be a corrective emotional experience for a particular patient, can we match the patient with a therapist who will facilitate this?

Negative Fit

The obverse of a corrective emotional experience may easily occur. It often arises from a negative fit between therapist and patient. Whereas such an outcome is particularly damaging to the morale of the beginning therapist, the experienced therapist may have equal difficulty in recognising when this process is happening, and be unable significantly to alter the nature of interaction (Colson, Lewis and Horwitz, 1985; Strupp and Hadley, 1985).

It was Luborsky and colleagues who described this important clinical phenomenon (Luborsky et al., 1971). It refers to the degree to which the therapist actually acts in ways that fit the patient's negative preconceptions (fears and expectations) about how people who have been important to him or her have responded to him or her. In a clinical study, L. Luborsky and B. Singer (1974, unpublished data) demonstrated two major patterns of negative fit in the tape-recordings of experienced therapists. One pattern was confirming the patient's fear of rejection by being critical, disapproving, cold, detached and indifferent, and the other was confirming the patient's fear of being made weak by being too directive, controlling and domineering. Bloomfield (1985, p. 303) points to the way in which the 'analyst is under pressure to fulfil a certain role in a scenario of which the patient – or rather patient's unconscious – is author–producer'.

It is often extremely difficult for the supervisor to discern that negative fit is occurring. The therapist will be aware, on some level, that all is not going well, but may only signal this in quiet asides, remarks made as the supervision ends, or by not coming to supervision when the difficulties are at their height.

The Nottingham Programme for Beginning Therapists

The Nottingham Psychotherapy Unit was established in 1974 and teaches at three levels, namely student, qualified health care professionals with a generalist interest in the subject, and career psychotherapists.

This paper focuses on the middle group, who have no previous experience of formal psychotherapy and who may, indeed, discover that what they have embarked on is not where their talents lie; the majority are stimulated to learn more.

Given the theory that I have outlined, what steps do we take to (1) prepare mainly inexperienced therapists for their role, and (2) work productively with interpersonal patterns that could lead to a positive or negative fit? Though the interpersonal perspective is by no means the only one taught in Nottingham, there is a general emphasis on teaching trainees to observe the relationship patterns that develop in therapy, to attend especially to awkward moments, to explore what they mean, and then work towards more fruitful patterns.

In this National Health Service Unit it is the 'walking wounded' who are referred, rather than the 'worried well'; these patients often have great potential for creating schizoid, paranoid and dependent attachment patterns. Thus, the cases are not as easy as they might be. Therapy is of the once-a-week, face-to-face variety and is open-ended in duration, though cases seen by beginners will generally be for a year to 18 months. Sessions are tape-recorded for the purposes of supervision, which is carried out in multidisciplinary seminars. It is important to note that the psychiatrist trainees are not formally selected by us; within the institution of the hospital we have to fulfil the requirement for psychotherapy teaching for psychiatrists in training made by the Royal College of Psychiatrists. With the others, if the applicant is not known to us, an informal assessment is made by a staff member.

The training sequence is as follows: beginning therapists join the introductory psychotherapy year, a weekly seminar which provides in the first 6 months an introduction to theory through guided readings, and to practise through role-play. After evaluation by the year leaders, the trainees take on selected Level I Psychotherapy Unit patients in individual therapy. In the second and subsequent years, trainees may join one of six supervision seminars, each with four members. The supervision experience may be extended by joining the reading seminar, and greater personal awareness gained through membership of the group course, the experiential group or personal therapy. At the end of each supervisory year, the supervisees and supervisors write structured evaluations of each other's psychotherapy work. Trainees seeing two or more patients may negotiate individual supervision.

Details are given of three aspects of the programme: (1) role-plays, (2) the written evaluation and (3) matching patient and therapist.

Role-plays

For many years, the ability of the beginning therapist to relate productively was honed through discussing video-tapes of patient interviews made by the trainee. In the last 18 months we have had a great deal of success with a role-play approach borrowed from the Manchester Psychotherapy Unit, and which is based on the work of Kagan. The seminar leader selects from a series of progressively more difficult, but commonly and usually fearfully encountered, problematic situations in psychotherapy. A secret instruction is given to either therapist or patient and the action allowed to unfold over a few minutes. At any stage the action may be halted to explore what one or other participant is feeling, what the group is obvserving and then, with greater awareness and confidence, the action is continued, repeated or moves in a new direction.

In the basic therapeutic skills set, examples of role-plays are insistently maintaining eye contact, stating repeatedly that you do not understand what is happening, and being surprised about everything. The second set deals with basic negotiating skills where examples are having the therapist practise telling the patient that a holiday break is coming up, or dealing with a request from the patient to increase the number of sessions per week. The third set entitled 'Misinterpretations in therapy' are dual-experience scenarios. Either party may be instructed to be suspicious of what is said, or to comment neutrally on the way the other is dressed. In the final set, graphically called 'Dealing with nightmares', fears of being seduced, engulfed, rejected or attacked are addressed. The patient's instruction may be to feel unattractive and tell the therapist that he or she is deliberately avoiding touching the patient, and express a wish for the therapist to disprove this, or undramatically to state that he or she has decided to kill him- or herself, or talk of impulses to smash up the room.

These role-plays are powerful, varied introductions to situations that all experienced therapists have faced. They allow the beginning therapist to work partially through his or her anxieties in the safer setting of the seminar, where fears can be anticipated, defensive strategies explicated and positive interventions practised.

Written evaluations

After 6 months into each supervisory year, seminar members and supervisors are expected to exchange informal evaluations, which 4 months later are the basis of written structured evaluations. The evaluations are confidential to that supervisory group, but a copy is held by myself as Organiser of Training. Some latitude is allowed in the way in which both parties complete the evaluations and discuss them in the group, but a number of headings are suggested. In the evaluation of the trainee, a brief description of the patients seen, their number, degree of difficulties and psychodynamics is asked for. The major section is on psychotherapeutic ability, under the headings of ability to form and sustain empathic relationships, handling of countertransference, conceptual ability, theoretical knowledge and other aspects. There are also headings for time-keeping with patient and in supervision, relationship with other members of the seminar and the supervisor, assets and weaknesses of the therapist and, finally, recommendations for further training.

Completing the evaluation is a taxing but rewarding task. The exchange of views is generally experienced as being constructive and a reflection of the professional attitude that the Unit takes to training. I also use written evaluations in the training of group therapists (see Chapter 14).

Matching patient and therapist

The literature on the therapeutic value of matching patient and therapist is inconclusive. Matching for socioeconomic status is one of the few consistently positive findings, with the benefits of matching for age and marital status being inconsistent (Berzins, 1977). Much more subtle attention needs to be paid to the interactive meaning of the dyad that can be gained from the crude alignment of demographic features. An intriguing study by Howard, Orlinsky and Hill (1970) showed that, when the therapist was an older married woman, her young married female clients reacted negatively, but young single female clients reacted positively. One can speculate that the latter fell more easily into a mother–daughter relationship, whereas with the former an element of competitive rivalry entered the picture.

Our clinical experience suggests some rules of thumb for matching patient and therapist. The validity of these 'rules' needs to be tested in sophisticated research studies. Assuming that the trainees have an ethical, affirmative and interested stance:

1. Encourage parataxic distortion by having the same sex therapist as the patient's major conflictual figure (age of therapist may be a major significant variable).
2. If the intrapsychic conflict is too severe, discourage parataxic distortion by having a therapist of the opposite sex to the patient's major conflictual figure.
3. Pair the patient with a therapist who has successfully resolved a similar conflict.
4. Avoid pairings where the therapist has similar conflicts to the patient and has been unable to resolve them.
5. Pair with the therapist who may complete the patient's negative pattern, but where this danger is judged to be amenable to being worked with.
6. Avoid unworkable, negative pairings.

Experienced therapists, if they are wise, tend to select patients with whom they can productively engage. Beginning therapists, if left to their own devices, will frequently choose patients whose conflicts are too similar to their own (see rule 4). The supervisor and the training institution have the responsibility of helping the trainee make a felicitous choice. For this to be more than guesswork, detailed knowledge of both members of the proposed dyad is required. Strupp and Binder (1984) have proposed an excellent formula to delineate the focal narrative of the patient. I see no reason why a similar analysis should not be applied to the therapist. In Nottingham, we have not taken such a step, but we are considering it.

A Damaging Interactive Dyad

This dyad is an example *in retrospect* of us trying to be too clever and attempting the difficult combination outlined in rule 5. With hindsight one can see that there were errors in assessment of both patient and therapist, though the pairing held out a possibility of beneficial learning for both. Though space does not allow me to develop the argument, I contend that developing a degree of negative fit is a necessary stage in successful therapy, as it is at that moment that the patient's self-destructive story becomes alive in the here-and-now of the therapy relationship. What distinguishes a successful therapy from an unsuccessful one is the skill of the therapist in recognising what is happening, and in working towards a different end (see Chapter 2).

The patient, a separated woman in her late twenties, had initially been offered group therapy to help overcome her lack of self-confidence and her passivity. In the event, she opted for individual therapy and was the first case for a male therapist, also in his twenties. In character, he presented somewhat arrogantly, chauvinistically, and had a take-it-or-leave-it style of interaction. His lack of sensitivity to the effect that he had upon others and a certain self-centredness made the leaders of the introductory year reluctant to have him take on a patient at the same time as his fellow course members. It was suggested that he might participate in the discussions in a supervision seminar, but delay taking a case. After a few months, his eagerness to advance his psychotherapy training and the flexibility that he had shown in the seminar encouraged his supervisor to allocate him a patient.

The patient's pattern was to undervalue herself and defer to the authority of others, particularly so with men. She was unable to pursue an autonomous path, and while she had talents and ability, would typically relinquish these as she entered into a new relationship with a man. It was anticipated that this pattern of passivity–dominance would be recreated in her therapy, *but* that (1) she could be helped by the therapist to assert herself, and (2) the supervisor could help the therapist accept her challenge and take a less dominant role.

What happened was that the therapist dominated the patient and she was unable confidently to challenge him. When this was pointed out, he would ask the patient if she felt dominated, but in such a way that she ended up apologising to him. This replicated another important element in her history: as a child, she had had to have numerous orthopaedic operations and was subject to a great deal of protective over-concern by her parents. More importantly, the home atmosphere was one of critical worry. Her parents took over and spoke for her; they appeared critical but felt they should not be critical. She felt that her mother had never been pleased with her, but it was impossible to voice this with her as her mother would become upset and retreat to bed, leaving the daughter feeling guilty.

In therapy it was difficult for the therapist to refrain from dominating her, but it was even more difficult for him to consider that the quality of interaction was damaging; he feared feeling inadequate. The pattern continued in the second year of supervision, with a different supervisor whose comments he had difficulty in hearing. He entered personal therapy but the point was reached when it was in the interests of both to stop the therapy. This was a difficult decision to reach and implement. In the termination period of six sessions, the hazard with the patient was that she would end therapy feeling that it had been yet another failure where she had been at fault, and with the therapist that the outcome would trigger a damaging sense of inadequacy, particularly as at that time the therapist's adequacy was being questioned in other quarters. We have some evidence that these hazards were avoided.

This case illustrates how, even with careful assessment and preparation, the voyage that we launch our patients and trainee therapists on may prove to be much more hazardous than we thought. It is important to state that, whilst the patient showed herself to be more damaged than was initially apparent, our view is still that she could gain from therapy *and* that the therapist has something useful to give to a patient with a different set of interpersonal problems. The patient will enter therapy with a different therapist and the therapist has an opportunity to join a new supervisory group and start with a new patient. How these stories will end awaits another telling.

References

ALEXANDER, F. and FRENCH, T.M. (1946). *Psychoanalysis Therapy: Principles and Applications.* New York: Ronald Press.

BERZINS, J.I. (1977). Therapist–patient matching. In: A.S. Gurman and A.M. Razin (Eds) *Effective Psychotherapy.* Oxford: Pergamon Press.

BLOOMFIELD, O.H.D. (1985). Psychoanalytic supervision – an overview. *International Review of Psycho-analysis* **12**, 401–409.

BLOUNT, C.M. and GLENWICK, D. (1982). A developmental model of supervision. APA Symposium on Psychotherapy Supervision: Expanding Conceptual Models and Clinical Practice, Washington DC.

BOHN, M. (1965). Counselor behaviour as a function of counselor dominance, counselor experience and client type. *Journal of Counseling Psychology* **12**, 346–352.

COLSON, D., LEWIS, L. and HORWITZ, L. (1985). Negative outcome in psychotherapy and psychoanalysis. In: D.T. Mays and C.M. Franks (Eds) *Negative Outcome in Psychotherapy*. New York: Springer.

COOPER, A. and WITENBERG, E.G. (1984). Stimulation of curiosity in the supervisory process. In: L. Caligor, P.M. Bromberg and J.D. Meltzer (Eds) *Clinical Perspectives on the Supervision of Psychoanalysis and Psychotherapy*. New York: Plenum Press.

HELLER, K., MYERS, R.A. and KLINE, L. (1963). Interviewer behaviour as a function of standardised client roles. *Journal of Consulting Psychology* **27**, 117–122.

HESS, A.K. (1986). Growth in supervision: stages of supervisee and supervisor development. In: F.W. Kaslow (Ed.) *Supervision and Training: Models, Dilemmas, Challenges*. New York: Haworth Press.

HOWARD, K.I., ORLINSKY, D.E. and HILL, J.A. (1970). Patients' satisfactions in psychotherapy as a function of patient–therapist pairing. *Psychotherapy: Theory, Research and Practice* **7**, 130–134.

LUBORSKY, L., CHANDLER, M., AUERBACH, A., COHEN, J. and BACHRACH, H.M. (1971). Factors influencing the outcome of psychotherapy: a review of quantitative research. *Psychological Bulletin* **75**, 145–185.

RACKER, H. (1968). *Transference and Counter-Transference* New York: International Universities Press.

SCHAFER, R. (1983). *The Analytic Attitude*. London: Hogarth Press.

STRUPP, H.H. and BINDER, J.L. (1984). *A Guide to Time-Limited Dynamic Psychotherapy*. New York: Basic Books.

STRUPP, H.H. and HADLEY, S.W. (1985). Negative effects and their determinants. In: D.T. Mays and C.M. Franks (Eds) *Negative Outcome in Psychotherapy*. New York: Springer.

STRUPP, H.H., HADLEY, S.W. and GOMES-SCHWARTZ, B. (1977). *Psychotherapy for Better or Worse*. New York: Jason Aronson.

SULLIVAN, H.H. (1970). *The Psychiatric Interview*. New York: W.W. Norton; Oxford: Pergamon Press.

Chapter 5
Psychotherapy: A Fundamental Discipline but an Academic Orphan

In this presentation, I discuss three related areas: first, the nature of formal psychotherapy and the way in which it may be perceived by academic colleagues and others; secondly, the potentially ambivalent relationship between psychotherapy units and academic departments; and thirdly, the urgent need for a greater commitment to psychotherapy by the academic world, a commitment which would go a long way towards resolving the catch 22 that many psychotherapists – and certainly those of a dynamic or interpersonal persuasion – find themselves in. I speak as a member of the Association of University Teachers of Psychiatry (AUTP) and a full-time NHS Consultant Psychotherapist, who has for 12 years been developing a new psychotherapy teaching and clinical service in the busy city of Nottingham, with its new medical school.

My ambition is to see the theory and practice of psychotherapy refined trough the enquiring, scholarly perspective, without detracting from the essential concern of psychotherapy with the individual and his or her experience and the nature and experience of his or her problematic social system. I would like to see academic psychiatry lending its weight to developing this aspect of psychiatric practice. A fruitful union could be made between practising psychotherapists and academics. Otherwise the present situation will continue, where the favourite children in the family psychiatric have their bowls filled, but not psychotherapy, a sibling born at the same time as his – or perhaps I should say her – brother, organic psychiatry. As has happened, psychotherapy, now substantially grown, will leave home and set up at a distance or, worse still, in opposition to the established order.

From M.O. Aveline (1986) Psychotherapy: A fundamental discipline but an academic orphan. *AUTP Newsletter* Winter, 9–14.

This was originally from a presentation at the AUTP conference on the relationship between the NHS and academic psychiatry, 31 October 1986, London.

The Nature of Psychotherapy and its Professional Image in the NHS

Practising psychotherapy is what many young entrants to psychiatry imagine their work will be. They enter with the idea that understanding what the patient feels, how and why he or she has arrived at this point in life, and what may be done to resolve the impasse, will constitute the focus of the professional role. All too often, the trainee is taught the more distant, more diagnostic stance which categorises symptoms into syndromes and disease processes, and which does not suggest that meaning is to be found in a person's experience. The concept of disease is preferred to that of dis-ease. The individual is seen as a representative of one or other collectives – hypomania or psychotic depression for example – whose presence predicates certain treatments. It is not my purpose to deny the validity of this approach – my medical training has acquainted me with the reality of organically based psychological disturbance, and I appreciate the arguments in favour of psychiatrists having a consistent language through which they can communicate their findings – but rather to emphasise the different perspective of psychotherapy.

All patients need to be approached with respect, compassion and understanding. Some patients will want to change the contribution that they make to their difficulties in life; they are candidates for formal psychotherapy, certainly for dynamic psychotherapy. Formal psychotherapy provides a structured, professional relationship in which the patient can learn to modify those learnt aspects of his or her nature that contribute to the present difficulties in relationships. The resolution requires careful, sustained effort by patient and therapist alike. I take the view that every person is, to a substantial extent, the author of his or her interpersonal fate. Those who seek psychotherapy have been encouraged to write, and have written sad stories for themselves. The skill of the psychotherapist lies in his or her ability to help them write new, more fruitful chapters in a book of sad endings. It is, as Freud termed it, a process of 'after education'. In my interpersonal model of psychotherapy – and here I acknowledge my debt to Harry Stack Sullivan – the patient is responsible for his or her actions and has a choice about the future: he or she is not the passive pawn of deterministic forces from the past. All this requires the most careful attention to what characteristically happens in the interactional sequence of the patient's problematic relationships, their replication within the consulting room, and the meaning that is placed upon these interactions and which in turn initiates their repetition.

All patients wish to be understood; not all wish to understand themselves and be responsible for their lives. All psychiatrists need to develop their skills as understanders; only a minority will wish to make this their life's work (Aveline, 1982). Without psychotherapy, psychiatry loses its heart and is a non-discipline (Aveline, 1984; see Chapter 1). Yet when we survey the psychiatric scene, we see general professional training schemes for psychiatrists struggling to implement the recommendations for psychotherapy that were laid down in 1971 (Royal College of Psychiatrists, 1971, revised 1986), a national provision of consultant psychotherapists that is only half-way towards fulfilling the College norms (Royal College of Psychiatrists. 1975) for teaching districts, and several regions with no consultant psychotherapist at all. In contrast, outside the NHS private training institutes proliferate, and without any academic scrutiny devise courses which may be inappropriate for NHS practice, or below the standards required. In the academic world, there is only a single Professor of Psychotherapy (in 1990 Digby Tantam was appointed to the first Chair of Psychotherapy at the University of Warwick). A Chair in Aberdeen was advertised but was unable to attract a candidate of sufficient academic achievement, and has now been shelved for a few years. At University College London, there is a special Professor, the Freud Professor of Psychoanalysis, a position held with distinction by Joseph Sandler, but this is not the same as a properly constituted academic department. A clutch of senior lecturers in psychotherapy in departments of psychiatry, less than five in total, completes the picture.

One reason for this is the poor professional image that psychotherapists have. They are often seen, I suspect, as other-worldly people who try hard but are rather ineffectual, or as elitists massaging the tender sensibilities of the middle class, or as touchy mysterious figures with arcane untested practices. The misperception that psychotherapists have an easy life just talking with the worried well, rather than, as I see it, struggling not to reinforce the self-destructive patterns of the walking wounded, arouses envy. The enormous difficulty of deciding upon and developing appropriate outcome measures in psychotherapy, and the way in which concepts such as unconscious motivation appear to be untestable and idiosyncratic in their interpretation, leads to a negative perception of the subject; ineffective, unscientific and imprecise are the adjectives that arise in the sceptical mind.

Negative perceptions foster the catch 22 of psychotherapy: if there is little of value to discover in the subject, it is not worth investigating; if the subject is not investigated, nothing will be discovered. One resolution to this self-perpetuating situation is to establish several proper academic departments of psychotherapy.

Of course, psychotherapists have contributed to this by practising behind closed doors, by being reluctant to record and make available for study what passes in the therapy hour, by being precious about

what they do, by interpreting criticism rather than explaining practices, and generally by being temperamentally unsuited to the cut and
thrust that the more directive, assertive members of the family psychiatric are so adept in. In what often feels like a hostile environment,
psychotherapists are prone to retreat into their units, where at least the
faciliatative environment for the practice of psychotherapy can be created. In so doing, physical form is given to division and opportunities
are curtailed for beneficial exchange between different, complementary viewpoints.

The Relationship Between Psychotherapy Units and Academic Departments

Teaching and research are the principal justifications for an academic
department. Psychotherapy units justify their existence by teaching
and clinical service. The two have teaching in common, and problems
may arise in this overlap. One academic colleague raised his eyebrows
when I described how between a third and a half of the working week
of members of staff in my unit went into teaching. Teaching was identified in his mind with didactic presentations, whereas in the psychotherapy world it largely means week-by-week supervision of
psychotherapy practice. In my unit, through 20 individual and 13 collective supervisory hours each week, we provide training in formal
psychotherapy for 61 therapists. In addition, on-site supervision in day-
hospitals, wards and the like provide support and skills development
for a further 42 therapists. We also provide around 3500 hours of
therapy each year for 180 new referrals. A similar work pattern is
recommended in the guidelines for the job descriptions of consultant
psychotherapists (Royal College of Psychiatrists, 1985): five sessions
should be for teaching, four for clinical service and the remainder for
research.

For the trainee, being committed to therapeutic work with a patient,
a couple, a group or a family over an extended period of time is a
valuable counterbalance to the hit-and-run mentality fostered by our
well-meaning desire as training organisers to fit as many postings as
possible into the 3-year period of general professional training in psychiatry. Full use can be made of the psychotherapist's ability to teach
trainees how to maintain, for most patients, a steady, containing, but
sufficiently challenging, therapeutic environment which will facilitate
self-reflection and personal change.

Teaching, however, may be seen to be the preserve of the academic
department. Territorial concerns can lead to resentment or jealousy.
This is more likely if the academic department or the psychotherapy
unit teaches a model of humankind that excludes the perspective of the

other or, through the mechanisms of splitting and projection, gets caught up in denigrating the other. I hope that we could be natural allies.

The individualistic perspective of psychotherapy is the antithesis of the collective perspective which dominates orthodox British psychiatry. In the former, all that is unique about a person and his or her history is brought into focus; in the latter, it is what that person has in common with others with similar symptoms that is stressed. It is easy for one approach to be subversive of the other.

My own commitment has first and foremost been to psychiatry. My goal – a grandiose one at that – is to encourage the development of a psychotherapeutically informed psychiatry. I feel that NHS psychotherapy should make its greatest effort with the severely personality disturbed – the schizoid, paranoid and dependent patients who tend to end up with psychiatrists. And yet, as I shall describe, it is this group, so destructive of themselves and to others, that psychotherapy is least effective with. A psychotherapy unit has to have its own identity and will need accommodation, essentially of a domestic type, to do its work well, but I have no wish to separate off from psychiatry. Such a move would impoverish us both, but I know that some of my colleagues do not share this view.

Research in Psychotherapy

Two points can be made:

1. Despite the voluminous research and descriptive literature in psychotherapy, no coherent comprehensive model exists of how people change. The models we have – insight, cognitive, behavioural and systems – are partial explanations, or are expressed in language which is mutually contradictory.
2. We lack the means to help the most personality damaged who are the most in need. Here is a twin challenge for the academic world to engage in. Limited time permits me only to explore the second. By sketching out two interesting recent research findings, I hope to indicate the parameters of one area which could be explored, given enough resources and time.

Hans Strupp and his colleagues at Vanderbilt University, as part of their development of an improved form of interpersonal psychotherapy (Strupp and Binder, 1984), have conducted a fascinating comparison of therapy conducted by friendly professors and experienced professional therapists; the friendly professors had no formal training in psychotherapy, but were chosen on the basis of their ability to interact comfortably with college students with personal problems.

Each met with their allocated patients individually, twice a week, for up to 25 hours; the patients were socially withdrawn and had clinically significant depression or anxiety. Overall, both sets of therapists achieved comparably good results, but within the patient–therapist dyads there was considerable variation. Experienced therapists did especially well with patients who were able to make maximum use of the traditional therapy relationship they were offered. Neither the friendly professors nor the experienced professors were notably effective in treating patients with pervasive personality problems, especially those of pronounced hostility, pervasive mistrust, negativism, inflexibility and antisocial tendencies, the type of patient who in my experience constitutes a significant proportion of referrals to an NHS psychotherapy unit.

The poor-outcome patients were difficult, awkward people who quickly evoked negative countertransference in their therapists. The failing therapeutic alliance was obvious from early sessions and certainly by session three, and was not significantly improved in the course of therapy. The negative countertransference was not contained and its expression through coldness, distancing and criticism probably reinforced the patients' poor self-image.

These, then, are the most difficult patients to treat successfully, but equally they are the most in need of help. Training had helped the therapists do especially well with patients who 'fitted' their model, but could not provide any effective remedy for a deteriorating therapeutic relationship. Put another way, the therapists in the poor outcome group were working at the limit of human benevolence and beyond. What to do at the limit of benevolence is an important practical question for therapists.

Similar findings have been reported by Colson, Lewis and Horwitz (1985) in an analysis of a subset of the famous Menninger Foundation Psychotherapy Research Project. Once more, patients with good outcomes were compared with those with poor outcomes. In the poor-outcome group there was a relative absence of a cooperative collaborative alliance between therapist and patient. Indeed, these patients were either elusive, dishooest and withholding in therapy, or angry and demanding in a near-psychotic way.

The poor outcome was a function of three factors. In the first place, although the patients appeared at assessment to have a relatively good level of interpersonal functioning, major personality disturbance of the borderline type emerged during therapy. In the second place, a negative countertransference was evoked, was perhaps recognised by the therapist, but was certainly not resolved and led to the breakdown of the therapy relationship in the same way that the personal relationships of the patient had failed in the past. A third, new factor was identified.

The families of these patients colluded with the negative patterns and undermined healthy behaviour in the patients. They encouraged hostile dependence and self-destructive action.

The difficulties that I have described could be advantageously explored through single case studies. There is a need to refine our ability to appraise the difficulties that a particular patient would pose in therapy. Better ways of handling negative countertransference must be found, so that a therapeutic alliance can be sustained. We need to look beyond the confines of the consulting room and see how the social system reinforces negative patterns, and find ways of altering that system if we are to have any success with people whose lives are so impoverished and who, inevitably, will create disturbance in others.

Conclusion

Psychotherapy is a fundamental discipline in psychiatry, but its importance has still to be recognised by the establishment of professorial departments of psychotherapy. A complementary relationship is possible with academic departments as long as each recognises and values what the other has to offer. In the NHS, special academic attention needs to be given to elucidating the processes of psychological change, especially in those patients with severe personality disturbance. For psychotherapists, they represent the greatest challenge. In their care, we could do with all the help that we can get.

References

AVELINE, M.O. (1982). The MRCPsych examination: time for change? *Bulletin of the Royal College of Psychiatrists* 6, 170–171.

AVELINE, M.O. (1984). What price psychiatry without psychotherapy? *The Lancet* 2, 856–859.

COLSON, D., LEWIS, L. and HORWITZ, L. (1985). Negative outcome in psychotherapy and psychoanalysis. In: D.T. Mays and C.M. Franks (Eds) *Negative Outcome in Pychotherapy and What To Do About It*. Chapter 3, pp. 59–75. New York: Springer.

ROYAL COLLEGE OF PSYCHIATRISTS (1971). Guidelines for training of general psychiatrists in psychotherapy. *British Journal of Psychiatry* 119, 555–557.

ROYAL COLLEGE OF PSYCHIATRISTS (1975). Norms for the staffing of a medical psychotherapy service. *Bulletin of the Royal College of Psychiatrists* October, p.4 and December, p.18.

ROYAL COLLEGE OF PSYCHIATRISTS (1985). Guidelines for regional advisers on consultant posts in psychotherapy. *Bulletin of the Royal College of Psychiatrists* 9, 40–42.

ROYAL COLLEGE OF PSYCHIATRISTS (1986). Guidelines for training of general psychiatrists in psychotherapy. *Bulletin of the Royal College of Psychiatrists* 10, 286–289.

STRUPP, H.J. and BINDER, J.L. (1984). *Psychotherapy in a New Key. A Guide to Time-Limited Psychotherapy*. New York: Basic Books.

Part II
Group Psychotherapy

Whereas family therapy is fashionable and individual therapy well established, group therapy is still a minority interest in psychotherapy circles. This is a regrettable state of affairs, as being a member of a cohesive purposeful group can be a uniquely encouraging experience in a person's life. In contrast to individual therapy, a group offers its members the opportunity to be altruistic and to discover that one can be of assistance to others with all the consequent benefit for self-esteem and what that implies. Groups present unlimited opportunities for interpersonal learning. In 'The group therapies in perspective', I compare and contrast key concepts in group analysis, encounter and the interpersonal, psychodramatic, gestalt and cognitive–behavioural approaches to group therapy. Since no one approach has all the answers, I highlight the strengths of each. However, in my view of all the approaches, the interpersonal approach captures what is most central to effective group psychotherapy. 'Interpersonal group psychotherapy', written with my Nottingham colleague Bernard Ratigan, describes the emphasis on 'here-and-now' learning and the existential concern with freedom, choice and responsibility. 'The practice of group psychotherapy with insulin-dependent diabetics' details the application of this form of group therapy by diabetologists in a research study of the value of an 11-session closed group.

My experience as a psychotherapist and trainer has taught me much about the internal and external pressures that bear upon the mental health professional. Brief groups, either as part of workshops, or training courses in group therapy, can provide a safe setting in which work and personal issues may be explored and some resolution achieved. Often such a group is the only place in a professional's life where personal tragedies can be disclosed, the burden of being a carer shared and the interprofessional stereotypical obstacles to being simply people together in a group overcome ('Personal themes from training

61

groups for health care professionals'). Leading such groups requires a high level of skill, energy and professionalism, especially if the duration of the group is brief. In 'Leadership in brief training groups for mental health care professionals', I offer guidance for good practice.

Chapter 6
The Group Therapies in Perspective*

Introduction

Jean-Paul Sartre's play *In Camera* was first staged in London in 1946. Two women and a man, all recently dead, are shown to a room by a polite but inscrutable valet who, having settled them in, retires and firmly closes the exit door, a door which to begin with they cannot open. This is Hell, a closed small group whose members have an eternity in which to torment each other with the truth about the nastier aspects of their personalities, truths which the protagonists initially try to avoid by neither speaking to nor looking at each other, but which are disclosed as soon as they interact, and in so doing, manifest the cowardliness, betrayals and narcissism artfully edited out in the initial tellings of their histories. They rend each other to the point where, towards the end, Garcin declares that 'Hell . . . is other people!'. However, earlier he has argued – futilely, as it turns out – that they could help each other by finding a spark of human feeling in themselves and having faith in the others, the only others left to them.

Sartre points to a bleak existential truth about the responsibility people have for the existence they have willed. On another level, the play could be read as a depiction of a therapy group gone wrong – a group that is cohesive, to be sure, and expert in exposing what is wrong, but has not learnt to comfort and heal. The valet as leader confines his role to holding the boundaries, a limited and limiting part. The result can be what happens in a therapy group, but it is a travesty of the positive collective strength that is there to be tapped in this

From M.O. Aveline (1990) The group therapies in perspective. *Free Associations* **19**, 77–101. (Published by Free Association Books, London.)

* Further examination of many of the topics in this review may be found in M. Aveline and W. Dryden (Eds) (1988) *Group Therapy in Britain*, Open University Press, Milton Keynes.

powerful, technically difficult and relatively neglected therapeutic modality.

As we come to the end of the 1980s, what common and divergent paths can be discerned in this way of working? Do some of the approaches have inherent advantages over the others, or provide a uniquely helpful perspective on group and individual process? Where is this approach to psychotherapy going, and what are some of the evaluative questions that need to be answered?

Before these questions can be tackled, the diversity of the group therapies has to be acknowledged. Groups may be (1) small (7–10 persons), medium (15–30 +) or large (30–70 +) in number; (2) open or closed in membership; (3) brief (8–16 sessions), medium (12–18 months) or long (3+ years) in duration; (4) single or mixed in sex, age range, ethnic background and problem; (5) stranger or therapeutic milieu and community in format; and (6) therapy, self-help, skills acquisition, educational or encounter in designation of purpose. Each major variant has its own – or many – explanatory conceptualisations of what is central in theory and consequent practice, which, of course, in actual practice is much modified by the exigencies of the situation and the personality and personal assumptions of the practitioner. In the arena of small-group therapy, the names group analysis, interpersonal, encounter, gestalt, psychodrama and cognitive–behavioural evoke their different parentages. What they have in common is a group (a minimum of five in number) made up of people who interact and influence each other in the hope that from their membership they will derive some special benefit for problems that have been framed, by and large, in interpersonal terms.

Origins and Key Concepts

In this section I indicate the historical and philosophical sources of the major forms of group therapy today. The account is focused on small-group therapies. In order to contain this review within reasonable bounds, only passing mention is made of the important group form of the therapeutic community, which has currently slipped from fashion, and of the dramatic expansion in self-help and single-sex groups, especially women's groups. The interpersonal approach, psychodrama, gestalt, systems, cognitive and learning therapy are reviewed before considering the contribution of psychoanalysis in the form of the Tavistock Model, group analysis and group focal conflict theory.

Of the founding fathers of psychotherapy, only Adler had a profound interest in group interaction and the way in which a group context may have a therapeutic effect. Despite the strong influence of psychoanalytic ideas on one school of group therapy (group analysis), the psychologies of Freud and Jung were intrapsychic in their focus and individual in their practice. It was Alfred Adler who asserted the principle of continuous action and reaction between the individual and the environment: no person is in isolation or stasis; every person is in the process of change and subject to community feeling. Where Freud looked back in time to causes of psychic processes, Adler looked forward to their goal, aim and intentionality. This led him to develop a briefer, more open and collaborative style of therapy in which other members of the patient's social system might, with their permission, be involved. He also originated therapeutic education in schools, which had as its central feature the bringing together of all the concerned parties in a problem and more – that is, mother, child, the involved teacher and fellow teachers and students of the method (Ellenberger, 1970).

Adler's *interpersonal* approach found its natural expression in Britain in 1938 when Joshua Bierer, a disciple, began the self-governing Social Therapeutic Club at Runwell Hospital. In Europe, Victor Frankl was one of his most distinguished pupils; his new teaching emphasised existentialism and the quest for purpose. In the USA Karen Horney, Erich Fromm and Harry Stack Sullivan all have an Adlerian emphasis, though each fails to give due credit to their originator. In linear descent from them comes the most eminent contemporary North American group therapist, Irving Yalom. His truly interpersonal group psychotherapy (Yalom, 1983, 1985) blends the interactive perspective of Sullivan and the vector psychology of Kurt Lewin with the warmth of the 'I–thou' encounter so movingly depicted by Martin Buber (1957) and Carl Rogers (1973) and the recognition of the importance of the ultimate existential concerns of meaning, purpose and death (Yalom, 1980; see Chapter 7). Responsibility, choice and personal change through the discovery and expression of hidden, more able social selves are key constructs.

I favour the interpersonal approach because of the emphasis on the transactional aspect of relationships. According to Sullivan (1953) and William James before him, the self is a social construct, formed out of the appraisals made by others. How someone is seen by others is how they see themselves. Individual sense of self-worth arises out of these appraisals and is maintained by security operations such as selective inattention. In interaction, individual needs may be responded to in a complementary or reciprocal way; depending on the nature of the need and the response, needs will be satisfied or frustrated and, consequently, the relationship will prosper or decay. Thus to illustrate these actions and reactions in turn, a child needs tenderness and the complementary response of tenderness from the mother if that need is to be met. Later in development, if the natural impetus towards activity and curiosity is not to be destroyed, the child's initiatives need to be responded to reciprocally by the parent making a facilitative space for the activity. Furthermore, all parties to a sequence of interaction are active participants in what happens; the aggressive person elicits complementary aggression or reciprocal submission from others; the person who can trust generally brings out trust in others, although occasionally the response is one of exploitation; what happens becomes the foundation for what happens next, and so on. This model provides a sequential framework which is well suited for the task of examining what happens in relationships between specific people. In therapy groups, individuals can come to see how they relate in complementary and reciprocal ways to different members and the consequences that follow and, with hard work, learn more fruitful and less fearful ways of being with their fellow humans.

From the interpersonal, we move to consider two therapists whose ideas are innovative in the field, but where a f.cus on interaction between members – in my view a cardinal feature of effective group therapy – has only latterly come to the fore.

It was again from Vienna, a prodigious centre for intellectual activity in the first three decades of this century, that another great personality in the history of group therapy came; his name was Jacob Levy Moreno. After studying philosophy and medicine he founded the Theatre of Spontaneity and then the therapeutic method of *psychodrama*, which seeks to resolve personally difficult situations through dramatisation and the release of creative forces inherent in the individual. The approach is intermittently group-orientated as the initial focus is with the protagonist, who is helped to realise – in the dramatic sense of the word – his conflicts; later, the audience, now in the role of group members, shares with the protagonist their own experience and associations to this tangible exploration of the inner world in which they have participated. The psychodrama provides a stage on which roles, counter-roles and potential roles can be experienced, and the associated feelings can be cathartically faced. Increasingly the method is used reflexively to examine the process of an ongoing group; thus it can be said to have come of age as a group therapy.

Fritz Perls, an analysand of Karen Horney and yet another innovator to take flight from the rise of National Socialism in Germany, was much influenced by Wilhelm Reich's interest in character armour and the meaning of body posture and tension, and Kurt Goldstein's work in gestalt psychology with the brain-damaged. The synthesis was gestalt therapy, which is fundamentally concerned with the way in which humans create meaning by singling out aspects of their experience from the rest, which then recedes into the background. In the gestalt world, therapeutic progress is achieved by making contact with what is out of awareness. The figure and the ground may be different aspects of the relationship that the individual has, either with himself or with others. In a group, myriad *Gestalten* form and re-form: member to member, member(s) to leader, and with the group as a whole; the different elements can be brought into focus by the leader and by group members as they become skilled in the approach.

Closely related to the complementary nature of gestalt formation is *systems theory*. Mention has already been made of Kurt Lewin, who in vector theory pointed to the influence of interpersonal forces on individual action and self-perception; in the 1940s he pioneered the educational use of T-groups (T for training) in the National Training Laboratories in the eastern United States, where the provision of a new social environment unfroze the individual from his or her past self-definitions and facilitated movement towards self-actualisation, a goal which Jung, less crassly, termed 'individuation'. Systems theory, which is derived from cybernetics, emphasises the interdependence of the constituent parts of the whole. Change in one part inevitably leads to change in others. Systems are organised hierarchically, and the product of the whole is greater than that of the parts. Healthy living systems are in a constant state of change and adaptation; in a group application, the task of the leader is to promote permeable boundaries which permit the free flow of communication between people as a prerequisite to adaptive change (Durkin, H.E., 1981; Durkin, J.E., 1981). The systems group therapist is concerned with equifinality, or the way in which events within the group initiate or block members' modes of interaction. As we shall see, a similar concept was earlier and separately developed in Britain by S.H. Foulkes with his ideas on group dynamics and the social matrix (Foulkes, 1948).

Before turning to psychoanalytic ideas, learning theory and the influence of cognition must be considered since they have much in common with the pragmatic, relatively ahistorical approach to learning about the self which is practised in the T-group. Ever since Dollard and Miller's (1950) attempt to understand analytic concepts such as repression, regression and displacement from the perspective of learning theory, and to show that behavioural techniques of modelling, the introduction of hierarchically arranged tasks and social reinforcement of successive approximations to goals were present in the analytical hour, there has been a modest amount of interest in exploring the overlap between these two major schools of psychoanalysis and behaviourism. However, to my regret, the dominant direction is of separate development, with both approaches being practised at least theoretically in pure culture. In *cognitive–behavioural* groups, the therapeutic gaze is firmly on finding solutions to real-life problems posed by the client members. Functional analysis of problematic

situations through the delineation of antecedents, behaviour and consequences, role rehearsal, the setting and review of homework assign-
ments and the analysis and challenging of negative cognitions and false
logic such as selective abstraction, overgeneralisation and personalisa-
tion (Beck et al., 1979) give a distinctive cast to this work. The leader
fosters a degree of group cohesiveness sufficient to facilitate the activities of the group, but the ever-present substrate of group process is
neither recognised nor explained; this is a considerable weakness in
the approach. Its strength is in the clear statement of goals and the
mechanism for achieving them.

It is to psychoanalysis that we now have to look for the most fruitful
source of ideas on the genesis of individual and group process. *Process*
refers to the way in which the fear underlying the factual focus and
content of the session moves the group as a whole or mobilises defensive strategies in the individual; it is the subtext that is there to be read
by anyone who knows the language.

I have left psychoanalysis till last not because I doubt its singular
importance for *all* group therapists as a conceptual framework, but because its concern has been intrapersonal rather than interpersonal; it has
therefore neglected the therapeutic force that is there to be awakened
between members. In the USA, the initially dominant classical school
transposed psychoanalysis into the public setting of the group (Parloff,
1967). This was therapy *in* the group with the leader working with one
member at a time, elucidating his or her past and present conflicts and
making intrapersonal interpretations; the leader's role was central, with
the non-active members being passive learners (Glassman and Wright,
1983). Slavson (1959) exemplifies this style. In contrast, analytical group
therapists – the British Institute of Group Analysis is the prime example –
work *with* the group and make use of its special properties; they clarify
unconscious group and individual processes, often with a historical
perspective. The interpersonal school integrates therapy *with* and *of* the
group, but with a here-and-now emphasis explicitly designed to mobilise
the ability of members to help each other.

Therapy *of* the group has been specially developed in Britain. The
treatment efforts of the leader are directed towards the group as a
whole and only minimally towards individual members; the aim is the
development of a healthy group which will of itself be the vehicle for
therapeutic change. In small groups, Bion (1961), first at Northfield and
later at the Tavistock Clinic, made pioneering observations about the
way in which groups collectively may avoid working in the therapeutic
sense of the word; his technique of group interpretation was further
refined by Ezriel. Their ideas live on in the Leicester Conference and
other educational events organised by the successful Tavistock Institute of Human Relations – which, despite their educational purpose

may, incidentally, have a therapeutic effect. A somewhat similar model of group process was developed by Whitaker and Lieberman (1964), but more of this later. Finally, the larger 'living and learning' group of the therapeutic community owes much to the innovations made by Maxwell Jones at Belmont Hospital (later renamed the Henderson Hospital) and subsequently at Dingleton, Tom Main at the Cassel, and David Clark at Fulbourn.

When one looks back at the degree of interaction between Bion and, later, Ezriel, and their group members, its sparsity is striking. To my mind, it is Bion as scientist studying the effects on a group of a relatively distant and immobile therapist who does not fully include within his view himself as participant in that which he is observing. The phenomenon of the group turning away from being a working group into the three basic assumption states of fight–flight, dependency and pairing exists, but the therapist's working style contributed to their genesis. As concepts, they are clinically useful but their simplistic appeal may all too readily lead beginning therapists to make them the mainstay of their practice.

Similarly, Ezriel's (1952) tripartite formulation of the group taking up a required relationship with him in order to not to fall into the avoided relationship for fear of that leading to a calamitous relationship in which the therapist is destroyed, retaliates or abandons the group, while analytically insightful and thought-provoking, had the effect of focusing the attention of the group on the therapist. In his role, he prided himself on being 'nothing but a passive projection screen except for his one active step of interpretation' (Ezriel, 1959) and was pleased that members perceived him as being unchanged – except, that is, for the biological features of ageing – during their years (up to 10) in the group. It must be said that members in this approach were largely unchanged too. Malan et al. (1976), in a meticulous follow-up study of outcome 2–14 years after termination from 2 or more years in consistently and expertly led groups at the Tavistock Clinic, found no evidence of effectiveness for this form of group treatment.

A preoccupation with group process appeared to have led to the neglect of the individual concerns which were the *raison d'être* of the group's formation, and which might have been remedied by greater warmth, open encouragement and participation in group interaction. Yet it is the analytic concepts of unconscious process moving the group as a whole, just as it does the individual and the mental mechanisms of splitting and projection, which have been particularly fruitful sources in understanding how and why a group process occurs. This understanding is not synonymous with effecting therapeutic change, but it is an essential element for the therapist, at least in well-informed group work, in comprehending what is happening.

Returning to the therapy *of* the group approach, S.H. Foulkes, a psychoanalyst who trained in Vienna, worked, like Bion, at the Northfield military rehabilitation centre during the Second World War. Whereas Bion, Ezriel and Sutherland were much influenced by object-relations theorists – Klein in the south and Fairbairn in the north – Foulkes was more influenced by Anna Freud's emphasis on ego functioning, and owed much to the field theory of Lewin and the gestalt psychology of Goldstein, to whom I have referred already. Bion and his co-workers developed the Tavistock Model, while Foulkes and his colleagues at the Maudsley Hospital and the Group Analytical Society, which he founded, evolved a distinctive transpersonal approach, that of group analysis. The Society's journal, *Group Analysis*, commenced publication in 1967 and the Institute of Group Analysis was established in 1971; the Institute plays an increasingly prominent role in professional group therapy in Britain, runs several introductory courses and offers a specialist training over 3–4 years (Pines, Hearst and Behr, 1982).

The central concept which Foulkes and his heirs elaborated is the *group matrix*. This refers to the web of communication and interrelationships that evolve in the group and form the common shared ground that determines the meaning and significance of events in the life of the group. Within the group (and in a person's life) the individual is seen as the *nodal point* of a social network which defines and shapes; in order to understand that person, one needs to consider the social context, the context which both forms the person and is formed by them, the ground that is background to their figure. Psychological disturbance is located between people, not in people in isolation. Neurotic people bring into the group the incompatibility between them and their original family group and recreate this by disturbed interpersonal processes with themselves at the focal point.

In group analysis, the communications of the group are viewed like the free associations of an analytic dyad. It is analytic thinking that underlies the useful concept of the *mirror reaction* whereby the individual reacts to repressed parts of himself present in others, usually by either attacking or protecting them. The potential to recognise and accept these aspects of self in others is a uniquely valuable feature of any form of group work, and in group analysis is a major fulcrum in bringing about therapeutic change. Other analytic concepts are those of *resonance*, where unconscious communication results in conflict-specific bonding between members who need each other for their complementary roles of dominant, submissive and the like (in passing, we may note that Harry Stack Sullivan, in his (1953) *Theorem of Reciprocal Emotion* (pp. 198–199), identifies this as a major process in the maintenance or decay of personal relationships); *polarization*, where the mental mechanism of splitting complex reactions leads to group members expressing the unresolved conflicts of some or one of their number through taking up contradictory, divergent attitudes or extruding the conflict through scapegoating; and finally the way in which shared deeply unconscious material is expressed in a loosening of group resistances through a chain of symbolic communications in the *condenser phenomenon*, whose common meaning can be understood only on subsequent reflection by the group.

Across the Atlantic in Chicago, ideas with a similar theoretical base were being developed independently (Whitaker, 1987). Both approaches drew on the work of Lewin and Goldstein; both contributed important conceptualisations of the group as a whole. Dorothy Stock (now Whitaker), Morton Lieberman and Roy Whitman were stimulated by the utility in defining individual dynamics of the nuclear conflict formula originated by their adviser, Thomas French (of Alexander and French (1946) fame). They devised *group focal conflict theory*. In their rich formula, the group as a whole is moved by shared themes which constitute a disturbing motive (wishes and impulses) that is in conflict with a reactive motive (fear or guilt). This is the group focal conflict. Thus far the formulation is a classic analytic one of impulse and anxiety – or, in Ezriel's terms, the avoided and calamitous relationships. The innovative contribution at the group level is that of the solution; solutions to the conflict may be either restrictive or enabling. The former alleviate the shared guilt or fear but leave the wish unacknowledged, unsatisfied and unexplorable (and equate to Ezriel's required relationship); the latter put members in touch with their fears and wishes, but in a climate of acceptance and the context of new forms of relationship. Successive solutions to the focal conflict(s) are the history of the group and form the group culture. This temporal and solution-finding emphasis represents for me a most positive aid for the leader in comprehending the sequence of developments in a particular group. It also indicates the way in which a group may collectively move forward to greater maturity and effectiveness.

Some Comparative Comments

To begin where the previous section ended, it will be clear that there is much overlap of perspective between the theory of group analysis and that of group focal conflict. Both are concerned with the group as a whole and, substantially, with the here-and-now of the group experience; neither takes it for granted that the group will automatically become a therapeutic place, and both charge the leader – or conductor, in group-analytic parlance – with partial responsibility for guiding the group towards greater awareness of the conflict which lies behind the symptom of disturbed communication in the group and the resolution of maladaptive (neurotic) patterns of relationship, evolved in the past and recreated in the present.

Two differences can be discerned. First, group analysis places greater stress, in achieving the aims of the group, on clarifying the communications that take place within the group matrix. As Foulkes said (1948, p. 169), 'working towards an ever more articulate form of communication is identical with the therapeutic process itself'. To my approval, greater emphasis is given in the group focal conflict approach to a corrective emotional experience in the group: 'for the neurotic patient, the therapeutic process involves the experience that the feared consequences [of recognising or expressing impulses] do not occur' (Whitaker and Lieberman, 1964, p. 163). Secondly, *resonance* in group focal conflict theory has a different connotation from that in group analysis; it refers to resonance between the prevailing group focal conflict and individual focal conflicts, the latter being nuclear conflicts which have been triggered by psychologically similar interactions in the temporal 'now' of the group. Of course, the group conflict is the associative product of one, several or even all the members of the group. In group analysis, resonance refers to the transference-determined conflict-specific bonding between members.

While accepting that the way an approach conceptualises the process of change may not be synonymous with the actual process, a comparison of this and of the members' and therapists' roles illustrates some significant differences. Let us begin with the leader. In group analysis, this role is relatively austere; he or she is the conductor who interprets the communications of the group and the social matrix, while staying in the background as far as possible and working towards the group taking responsibility for itself; he or she derives authority from the projections of the group, which are then used for the benefit of the group; he or she has an analytical love of the truth, even when it is unpalatable. The conductor does not aim to give comfort or be real. In contrast, the interpersonal leader is a fellow-traveller in the journey of life and construes the role as being a facilitator of interpersonal transactions. As in gestalt group therapy, the leader endeavours to present a model of good group membership through being open (but not irresponsibly so), taking risks and being relatively undefended. In gestalt, psychodrama and cognitive–behavioural group therapy, the therapist is definitely directive. The gestalt leader may initiate technical procedures and certainly acts to frustrate confluence and promote its antithesis, contact. For the leader in psychodrama, the role of director is prominent and responsible; analyst and producer are subsidiary roles. The director has the responsibility for selecting which protagonist to work with and then following the spontaneous cues given by that person through each stage of the drama to the very important twin end-point of de-roling and the audience sharing their experience. Success in the role of director requires an uncommon blend of extroversion and sensitivity as well as energy and the ability to think on one's feet and tolerate the scrutiny of the group. The cognitive–behavioural therapist takes the stage as educator; he or she may be didactic, directive, evaluative and, above all, flexible in modifying techniques to the needs of particular clients; he or she promotes the acquisition of skills.

The roles of conductor, facilitator, director and educator make their different appeal to each therapist. This fact needs to be recognised by trainees when they are selecting a training.

In contrast to the individual world of classical psychoanalysis, where insight is vertical along an axis reaching back from current relationships with the analyst and significant others into the patient's formative past (the there and then), effective group therapy takes place along the horizontal plane of the here and now of the group and the historical dimension is not essential. It is primarily in the here and now that members undertake their work of change. In both modern psychoanalysis and group psychotherapy, working with the here and now of the relationship is central to the process of effecting change.

In this artificially created social context, a member, from the perspective of group analysis, communicates his or her problem by the symptom of blocks to free communication; the member is at the nodal point of a network of disturbed communications whose meaning is initially unintelligible; interpretation clarifies the latent meaning, and members make progress as they give up their focus on the declared problems and enter into the ongoing life of the group. The conductor's adherence to boundaries, which has the effect of bringing transference issues into sharp focus, is an important element in the approach. The end result of maturation and individuation is similar to that of an interpersonal group. Here the member brings to the group his or her recurrent interpersonal difficulties and enacts them within it; the group forms a laboratory wherein maladaptive interactions can be identified, and a workshop where new resolutions may be practised. It is through the exercise of responsibility and choice that a sense of meaning and purpose in life is strengthened and the individual gains the courage to enter into the selves that they might have expressed had they been less fearful. In the analytic and the interpersonal group, although useful gains may be made in brief closed groups of 8–16 sessions or in intensive workshops over a few days, the characteristic mode is weekly or biweekly work over upwards of 18 months.

All group therapies require their members to be physically present and emotionally available, to be open to change and to have sufficient self-generated willingness to commit themselves to meeting and involving themselves in each other's cares. An ability to withstand the group process is a necessary qualification for all, and the ability to understand or work towards understanding the process is a prerequisite for groups that reflect on their evolving history; group-analytic, group focal conflict and interpersonal analytic groups certainly come into this category, as may gestalt and psychodrama groups led by process-minded therapists. Often – and this is an important limitation – gestalt and psychodrama groups are not reflexive; they meet episodically and, because of the focus on work with the individual, do not reflect on the significance of intermember and member–leader interaction.

Experimentation, creativity and catharsis are three elements in the process of change which are given full rein in psychodrama; these elements extend the roles which the individual has. By acting through the important roles that they and significant others in their cultural world take, fuller and warmer understanding of the roles and counter-roles is reached, old and avoided feelings are expressed and, selected from their cultural atom (the total range of roles open to that person), a more effective and fulfilling range of roles is acquired. The specific technique of role reversal may – but only may – increase tolerance of others and the acceptance of compromise.

Collusive restrictive patterns so well described in group focal conflict theory are recognised by interpersonal group therapists, and are addressed as such by psychodramatists who wait for a protagonist to come forward who will unknowingly be the spokesperson for the group anxiety, and by gestaltists in the resistance to contact between members which becomes the figure in the ground for the group. With the exception of cognitive–behavioural, all the approaches make use of psychoanalytic concepts such as transference or parataxic distortion, projection, splitting and mirroring.

In contrast to the other approaches, the cognitive–behavioural group is much more goal-directed in its focus and will rarely meet for more than 12 sessions. Symptom removal is given precedence over self-understanding. The purpose is to modify specific problematic cognitions and behaviours put forward by the client; these may or may not have an interpersonal cast. The clients are taught how to manage feelings of anxiety; how to improve social skills, which may have a secondary effect of improving interpersonal effectiveness; and how to use techniques for identifying, testing and modifying distress-inducing thoughts and beliefs.

Reference has already been made to the differential appeal to therapists of their varied role in each of the smaller-group therapies. The same is likely to be true for the group members. Foon (1987), in an interesting review of the research literature on Rotter's (1966) concept of locus of control as a predictor of outcome, reaches two relevant conclusions. First, she concludes that subjects whose locus is external – who tend, that is, to perceive their behaviour as determined by forces outside themselves, such as chance, fate and dictates of society – prefer directive behavioural approaches in therapy. In contrast, internals whose behaviour is seen as generated by themselves and where reinforcements follow causally, prefer non-directive analytic therapies. Secondly, outcome is improved when the control orientation of therapist, therapy and subject is the same. These conclusions have some face validity for group therapy. Certainly cognitive–behavioural group therapy and, in my experience, some forms of psychodrama and gestalt groups, are qualitatively different from analytic and interpersonal groups. In the former, the member is acted upon; in the latter, the member is engaged in a process of self-reflection. In both, a good therapy outcome may be marked by that person's locus moving more within him- or herself as he or she comes to feel and be more in charge of life.

The successful traverse of the above process depends on the willingness of a person to set him- or herself along one course out of many. As therapists, we need to consider carefully what our patients want from their group experience and how they may best achieve it. To single out three dimensions from many in helping the patient make an informed choice (I assume, idealistically, that a choice is available), control orientation is one, the intention of symptom removal or self-understanding another, and the special character of the different small-group therapies a third. By special character, I mean aspects of the group which have either the potential to make good individual deficiencies or an intrinsic appeal to a member's character. For example, when faced with an inhibited, serious person, I think how valuable a corrective might be the opportunity to play in psychodrama; conversely, the extrovert also does well in this medium. When issues of power and control threaten the establishment of a therapeutic alliance, the flattened power differential of the interpersonal group is particularly appropriate. When a person is seeking introspective answers and has sufficient personal resources to sustain him or her in the quest, my preference turns towards analytic groups.

Thus far this review has surveyed the historical and philosophical sources of the major forms of group therapy, especially small groups. It has detailed a number of key concepts used to understand the work of the group and compared conceptualisations of the members' and leader's roles. Some pointers have emerged towards matching a patient with the most suitable group. All this can be taken as a statement of intent, linked theoretically with outcome. We have not, however, discussed what mediates a therapeutic effect in groups. It is to this aspect that we now turn.

Therapeutic Factors in Group Therapy

In 1955 Corsini and Rosenberg factor-analysed elements identified in the literature by experienced group therapists of many persuasions, about what were the active ingredients in promoting personal change through group therapy. The resulting classification comprised nine fairly clear-cut factors and a tenth miscellaneous factor. Overall, the ten factors could be assigned to three broad categories – intellectual, emotional and actional. This work has provided a framework within which to investigate what happens in different groups at different stages of development, and helped to identify what group members particularly value in their experience. In addition to experimental, correlational and analogue studies, productive naturalistic studies have been carried out using either the methodology of the Q-sort – as in Yalom et al.'s classic 1968 study of 20 successful outcomes in long-term group therapy – or 'the most important event' for members in sessions (see Yalom, 1985). A refined classification is slowly emerging.

Bloch and Crouch (1985) identify ten factors whose relative importance is a function of the group's goals, size, composition, duration, stage of development and context. They define a *therapeutic factor* as an element of the group process which exerts a beneficial effect on group members; they distinguish this from a *condition for change* – which must be present for a therapeutic factor to operate, but does not have an intrinsic therapeutic effect – and a *technique*, which is a device available to the leader to promote the operation of therapeutic factors. The ten factors are: acceptance, universality, altruism, instillation of hope, guidance, vicarious learning, self-understanding, learning from interpersonal action, self-disclosure and catharsis.

Bloch and Crouch's factors overlap and are interdependent. Within the list, some are of cardinal importance and, as I have said, the relative importance varies with the type of group and its stage. Let us consider (1) the long-term group, (2) the effect of stage of development, (3) in-patient as opposed to out-patient groups, and (4) groups with the elderly.

At this point, I must declare again my bias towards interpersonal groups. I believe they distil out what is most helpful in brief, medium- and long-term groups which are designed to facilitate change in personal functioning through enhanced knowledge of self and others and the taking of new action. There is circularity in my bias, as self-knowledge and the taking of new action are central to my concept of what, in its essence, explorative individual and group psychotherapy have to offer in promoting personal change, and hence shape how I construe my task as therapist. Research evidence, though not conclusive, supports this position.

In Yalom's (1985) classic study, successful graduates of long-term group therapy (18-months plus) rank-ordered 64 questions about what had helped them most. The top three answers were 'Discovering and accepting previously unknown or unacceptable parts of myself',* 'Being able to say what was bothering me instead of holding it in', 'Other members honestly telling me what they think of me'. Comparable therapy groups have yielded similar research findings. In other words, the group forms a social microcosm in which once a sufficient degree of cohesiveness (acceptance) has developed, members may disclose with feeling matters of concern to them (self-disclosure and catharsis) and learn from their interaction with their fellow members, both about themselves in the here and now of the group and from new action undertaken in the group (self-understanding and learning from interpersonal action). Clearly, in achieving this level of working in the group, what has gone before in the early stages acts as the foundation for what is built later, and there is much reworking of themes. In this, disclosure and feedback are central, recurrent acts; they serve to reduce the façade presented by a member to the group, and illuminate blind spots. As members draw each other into their particular self-restricting patterns of interaction, the group is helped by the leader to reflect on what it has been caught up in,† the so-called reflective loop (see Chapter 7).

Whilst what group members value most may not be the same as what is actually helpful, the above findings must command our attention. I suggest that it behoves the leader in all forms of group therapy to foster interaction, group and individual reflection on the meaning and significance of past and present interactions within the group, and a climate of acceptance in which members can take risks, discover strengths and be of assistance to their fellows. These are cardinal therapeutic factors. I also believe that leaders need to have a professional knowledge of unconscious individual and group processes, as without this there will be no understanding of the individual and shared conflicts that impede the operation of the cardinal therapeutic factors in the group and must at times be addressed if the group is to work in the Bion sense of being a cooperative, lively, enquiring and purposeful entity. Although my

---

* The first answer has a North American feel to it but in content is similar to the statement by Sandler and Sandler (1983) that a major aim in psychoanalysis is 'to get the patient to become friends with previously unacceptable parts of himself, to get on good terms with previously threatening wishes and fantasies'. (Quoted in J. Sandler and A. Sandler (1983) The past unconscious, the present unconscious, and interpretation of the transference. *Psychoanalytic Inquiry* 4: 367–399.)

† A related concept is to be found in group analysis. Here, the individual will be at the nodal point of the group and will be communicating the nature of the disturbance through the group matrix.

view may not be shared by all, it is the cardinal therapeutic factors that bring about change in personal functioning; addressing process is a way, and often the only way, of liberating their operation. In other words, interpreting process is a means to an end; it is not an end in itself.

Groups pass through stages in development, though the order is by no means uniform or hierarchical. Schutz (1966) pithily characterises a common progression of concern with issues of membership ('in–out') to dominance ('top–bottom') and intimacy ('near–far'). Another facet of group life is change over time in members' needs and goals; usually this shifts from a narrow concern with symptom relief to a more funda-mental desire to alter interpersonal life. Early on in a group, members place great value on the instillation of hope, universality and guidance. In contrast, the longer members are in the group, the more they value the cardinal therapeutic factors outlined in the previous paragraph. One might say that once members sense that they can survive being in the group, and have confidence that the group will endure, then they are ready to learn.

In-patient groups have their own character. The leaders have less opportunity to select a balanced group, members are more likely to have major psychiatric illness, turnover is high, continuity of member-ship uncertain and boundaries blurred. Indeed, Yalom (1983, 1985) goes so far as to say that the leader should reckon the life of the group to be a single session. Hence he advocates an active, directive and open style of leadership, with effort put into fostering a supportive, con-structive atmosphere. In this structured session, the leader aims for achievable goals of engaging the patient in the therapeutic process, reducing anxiety about admission, problem-spotting and illustration in the here and now, decreasing isolation and enabling people to be help-ful to others. Roberts (1986) comments that the turnover of the in-patient population is less frenetic in the UK than in the USA, and that on wards here it is possible to run brief, modified analytic groups with limited goals. The research literature indicates that in this kind of group patients value universality, altruism, acceptance and, to a lesser extent, self-disclosure and insight.

In a welcome rejection of the early therapeutic pessimism about psy-chotherapy with people beyond their middle years, and perhaps as a response to the prevailing demographic shift into old age, group therapy is being undertaken with the elderly. Elderly people easily become disen-gaged and depressed. They suffer narcissistic losses in role and health, and face a future of declining gratifications. They are prone to identify with society's negative stereotype of old age. Leszcz et al. (1985), in an encouraging account of a group for male residents aged 70–95, stress the importance of universality, acceptance, learning from interaction and altruism. The group offers its members two uniquely helpful opportunities: the chance to reminisce and life-review. Reminiscence with peers and, in my experience, across generations when the leaders are much younger and appreciative of what they are hearing, reconnects the elderly person with lost ego-strengths and helps to restore a sense of personal value (Poulton and Strassberg, 1986).

The foregoing examples are not intended to be full expositions of how to work with different kinds of group, but rather to indicate that modifications in technique are necessary. The well-trained leader will have a depth of knowledge and experience in one form of group therapy, or at best, several forms. But in each therapy situation, be it stage or specialised form, three steps need to be taken: first, an assessment of clinical realities; second, a formulation of goals that are appropriate and achievable; third, the modification of technique and focus. This is on the macro-level. On the micro-level of the moment-to-moment interaction within the group, the leader, in considering whether or not, or how, to intervene, needs to consider both the individual and the collective, process and content, and the shared lived history of the group (see Chapter 13).

A Look to the Future

'Hell . . . is other people!', Garcin declared. Hell can be other people, but this is not inevitable. The images that each person forms of him- or herself, and of what may be expected from others, arise through interaction. It is in interaction that new views may be formed – not all of them flattering – and new possibilities discovered. Therapy groups can offer a rich opportunity for interaction with several others, each of whose experience of life and style of coping is different. Where one may be weak, another will be strong. Where one may be beginning, another may be some way down a similar path of personal difficulty, and can offer guidance and assistance with the unfamiliar terrain. These roles are not fixed but may alternate within sessions and over time. Groups provide the chance to be altruistic and discover that one can be of assistance to others, with all that that implies for improving an inner sense of low worth. Being a member of a cohesive, purposeful group may be a uniquely encouraging experience in a person's life.

Furthermore, no other treatment setting allows such opportunities for interpersonal learning through testing out how one is seen, how one's inner self may be received and what effects negative and positive acts have, and for recognising and undoing defensive strategies. The reactions of fellow members have great force, as they are seen as coming from unbiased peers and not from therapists who are compelled, professionally and financially, to be supportive. In the stranger group, risks in the form of new interaction may be taken which might be too disruptive to the natural group of the family and the marriage, or might be opposed by a dynamic wish in others to maintain the status quo. My emphasis here is on the benefit members can derive from peer inter-action, and the impression may have been created that the leader is a redundant figure in the group. This is far from the truth. The leader has an essential function in forming the group, holding its boundaries and fostering among the members a healthy culture of open, enquiring and respectful interaction and reflection on their dynamic processes.

Given all this, why is not group therapy the dominant modality in psychotherapy practice? Uncongeniality, difficulty and fashion are part answers. How these answers are addressed will shape the future of the group therapies.

It is not surprising that many patients find the prospect of being in a therapy group uncongenial. Most seekers after psychotherapy have a sense of their inner person being bruised, weak or unequal to the task of living. They fear, often to the point of phobia, the meeting with others which is central to group therapy. 'How can I disclose? How can I share?', they ask. Yet it is the most fearful persons who stand – if they can bear it – to gain most from this approach. Some, whose capacity to trust is very limited, may need individual therapy alone or as a first experience. All benefit from thorough pre-group preparation, the one intervention that is linked consistently with improved outcome in the research literature. I expect to see the development of more refined means of preparation.

Just as members find their time in the group difficult, so do leaders. The phenomenological field is vast, group process tumultuous in their impact and intervention decisions have to be made without the luxury of prolonged reflection. Historically and preferentially, the allure of individual therapy remains great. Trainees may better appreciate the special merits of group therapy if they have been members of a well-led training group and are well supervised in their first essay as leaders. These are points to do with the potentially discouraging effect on trainees of the inherent complexity of group therapy and the ameliorat-ing effect of good experiences as members and leaders of groups. A more fundamental point concerns what experience should lie at the heart of the training of group therapists in any of the described modes. Here, I advocate that the foundation experience as group leader be for 18 months in the analytic or interpersonal mode, as these approaches provide a rich conceptual framework for understanding the interper-sonal and group processes that are present in all groups, and which may be harnessed in the therapeutic service of the group. They provide a frame of reference against which special approaches learnt later in training may be deployed; the frame may or may not be explicitly referred to in practice, but is there to be drawn on in case of need (see

Chapter 13). To return to the opening theme of this paragraph, however, fashion in therapy practice may limit the availability of groups, and thereby restrict the number of entrants to the field.

Consider how fashion has affected the therapeutic community. The springs of this movement − for that is what it is − lie with Tuke's moral treatment at the beginning of the last century, and Lane's initiative in self-government for disturbed adolescents at the beginning of this. The Northfield experiment during the Second World War was a major historical landmark, but the movement as a radical, powerful force reached its apogee in the 1960s and early 1970s. Rapaport's well-known quartet of ideological tenets held by staff at the Henderson Hospital − democratisation, permissiveness, reality-confrontation and communalism − were in tune with social and political movements in the world at large, movements characterised by their anti-authoritarian, anti-psychiatry and pro-commune nature. This harmonisation fostered the growth of a wide range of therapeutic communities whose charismatic leaders articulated what a sufficient proportion of the people wanted to hear. Those days are past, as the new conformist but essentially self-centred ethic of 'me-first' and 'me having a right to a good personal relationship' has arisen, an ethic which is antithetical to Adler's concept of community feeling. Therapeutic communities continue, but in a less idealised, more modest form. Certainly, their principles will need to be understood if the establishment of day facilities and the like as part of the move to community psychiatry is to succeed.

What has seized the imagination of psychotherapists is direct work with families. Systems theory, by indicating the interdependence of the constituent parts and the possibility of influencing the system as a whole by working with its members, has provided a conceptual framework for intervention with the praxis that underlies much emotional disturbance. I anticipate that this form of therapy with naturally constituted groups will continue vigorously for some years, and will influence the practice of the subject of this review, stranger group therapy. There will be a greater emphasis in theory and practice on concepts derived from sociocultural and systems theory.

Two other developments are set to have a fair run: single-sex and self-help groups. Both are on the upward curve of their development. Single-sex groups have been fuelled by the women's movement, and the literature is largely by women about women. Perhaps as a reaction to this, and certainly given fresh impetus by the spread of AIDS, there is a complementary development of men's groups. The findings in women's groups are already leading to the development of a female psychology, less paternalistic than the present one. Issues of self-pride, support and competition among women and the intense, mutually ambivalent bond between mother and daughter are coming to the fore and are being explored in more informal and democratic groups, which provide some insulation from male dominance (Price, 1988). This format is likely to have drawbacks as well as benefits and, just as with any form of therapy, its claim to the therapeutic advantage must be tested (Huston, 1986).

Whatever the problem, it is likely that now there is a self-help group to which the sufferer and, often, non-afflicted family members can turn. If one does not exist, then the essence of the development is to set one up, drawing – if the founders so wish – on professional expertise (Wilson, 1986). While some of these groups work closely with medical and other formal services, many reject professional involvement as they see this leading to a damaging loss of independence. I regret the rejection, but simultaneously applaud the diversity of approach and the forum that such groups provide for positive self-action, non-professional support and good neighbourly care.

Finally, to return to stranger small-group therapies, I see a good future for this form for two reasons. First, it has special advantages for learning over individual therapy. Second, whilst one can often discern the process of the patient's problems in the praxis of his or her natural group, be it the family or the couple, the natural group may not be accessible or, more important, may be inimical to the change desired by the patient. For me, interpersonal and analytic groups, especially those informed by group focal conflict theory, have the most powerful model for promoting change in interpersonal functioning and understanding its process; their insights and practice will remain central. However, to advance the practice of small-group therapy much work needs to be done on translating the conceptual insights of one approach into the language of the others, and then seeing how unique insights and practices may or may not be integrated into the other without detriment to the pure culture practice. Positive examples that could be investigated are the emphasis on play and creativity in psychodrama, immediacy and non-intellectualisation in gestalt, and clarity of purpose and the value of experimentation through homework in cognitive–behavioural therapy. We must take account of research findings on therapeutic factors and investigate how to match optimally problem, patient and variant of group therapy. We must determine what can be achieved in a brief therapy group and what necessitates a long experience.

References

ALEXANDER, F. and FRENCH, T. (1946). *Psychoanalytic Therapy: Principles and Applications*. New York: Ronald Press.
BECK, A.T., RUSH, A., SHAW, B. and EMERY, G. (1979). *Cognitive Therapy of Depression*. New York: Guilford Press.

BION, W. (1961). *Experiences in Groups*. Tavistock.

BLOCH, S. and CROUCH, E. (1985). *Therapeutic Factors in Group Psychotherapy*. Oxford: Oxford University Press.

BUBER, M. (1957). *I and Thou*. New York: Scribner.

CORSINI, R. and ROSENBERG, B. (1955). Mechanisms of group therapy: processes and dynamics. *Journal of Abnormal and Social Psychology* **51**, 406–411.

DOLLARD, J. and MILLER, N.E. (1950). *Personality and Psychotherapy*. New York: McGraw-Hill.

DURKIN, H.E. (1981). The group therapies and general systems theory as an integrative structure. In J.E. Durkin (Ed.), *Living Groups: Group Psychotherapy and General Systems Theory*. New York: Brunner/Mazel.

DURKIN, J.E. (1981). Foundations of autonomous living structure. In: J.E. Durkin (Ed.) *Living Groups: Group Psychotherapy and General Systems Theory*. New York: Brunner/Mazel.

ELLENBERGER, H.F. (1970). *The Discovery of the Unconscious*. New York: Basic.

EZRIEL, H. (1952). Notes on psychoanalytic group therapy: II Interpretation and research. *Psychiatry* **15**, 119–126.

EZRIEL, H. (1959). The role of transference in psychoanalytic and other approaches to group treatment. *Acta Psychotherapeutica* **7**, 101–116.

FOON, A.E. (1987). Review: locus of control as a predictor of outcome of psychotherapy. *British Journal of Medical Psychology* **60**, 99–107.

FOULKES, S.H. (1948). *Introduction to Group-analytic Psychotherapy*. London: Heinemann.

GLASSMAN, S.M. and WRIGHT, T.L. (1983). In, with, and of the group A perspective on group psychotherapy. *Small Group Behaviour* **14**, 96–106.

HUSTON, K. (1986). A critical assessment of the efficacy of women's groups. *Psychotherapy* **23**, 283–290.

LESZCZ, M., FEIGENBAUM, E., SADAVOY, J. and ROBINSON, A. (1985). A men's group psychotherapy of elderly men. *International Journal of Group Psychotherapy* **35**, 177–196.

MALAN, D.H., BALFOUR, F.H., HOOD, V.G. and SHOOTER, A.M. (1976). Group psychotherapy. A long-term follow-up study. *Archives of General Psychiatry* **33**, 1303–1315.

PARLOFF, M.B. (1967). Advances in analytic group therapy. In: J. Marmor (Ed.) *Frontiers of Psychoanalysis*. New York: Basic.

PINES, M., HEARST, L.E. and BEHR, H.K. (1985). Group analysis (group analytic psychotherapy). In: G.M. Gazda and C.C. Thomas (Eds) *Basic Approaches to Group Psychotherapy and Group Counselling*. Springfield, Il: C.C. Thomas.

POULTON, J.L. and STRASSBERG, D.S. (1986). The therapeutic use of reminiscence. *International Journal of Group Psychotherapy* **36**, 381–397.

PRICE, J. (1988). Single-sex therapy groups. In: M. Aveline and W. Dryden (Eds) *Group Therapy in Britain*. Milton Keynes: Open University Press.

ROBERTS, J.P. (1986). Inpatient group psychotherapy. *British Journal of Hospital Medicine* **136**, 367–370.

ROGERS, C. (1973). *Encounter Groups*. Harmondsworth: Penguin.

ROTTER, J.B. (1966). Generalised expectancies for internal versus external control of reinforcement. *Psychological Monographs* **80**, 1–28.

SCHUTZ, W. (1966). *The Interpersonal Underworld*. Palto Alto, CA: Science and Behavior Books.

SLAVSON, S.R. (1959). *Analytic Group Therapy with Children, Adolescents and Adults*. New York: Columbia University Press.

SULLIVAN, H.S. (1953). *The Interpersonal Theory of Psychiatry*. London: W.W. Norton.

WHITAKER, D.S. (1987). Some connections between a group-conflict and a group-focal perspective. *International Journal of Group Psychotherapy* 37, 210–218.

WHITAKER, D.S. and LIEBERMAN, M.A. (1964). *Psychotherapy Through the Group Process*. New York: Atherton.

WILSON, J. (1986). *Self-help Groups: Getting Started, Keeping Going*. New York: Longman.

YALOM, I.D. (1980). *Existential Psychotherapy*. New York: Basic.

YALOM, I.D. (1983). *Impatient Group Psychotherapy*. New York: Basic.

YALOM, I.D. (1985). *The Theory and Practice of Group Psychotherapy*, 3rd edn. New York: Basic.

Chapter 7
Interpersonal Group Therapy*

Historical Context and Development in Britain

The origins of interpersonal group psychotherapy lie in an amalgam of German existential philosophy, American self-psychology and British analytic theory. Its practice is focused on what happens between people and how these interactions may be used to facilitate desired changes in maladaptive patterns of relationships. Although the personal histories of members are important, the work of the group is primarily with the here-and-now interactions within the sessions. Fundamentally, the approach is ahistorical. The group is both a laboratory where the form of interactions reveals the nature of the members' difficulties, and a workshop where new resolutions may be achieved and practised.

The central concern of psychoanalysis has been with intrapsychic processes; thus, the exploration of them characterises the practice of psychoanalytic psychotherapy and analytically inspired group therapy. In contrast, and at much the same period as when Freud was elucidating the workings of the unconscious, existential philosophers in Germany were exploring the ways in which humans define their own existence – their *Dasein* or being in the world – and through this, find meaning in their life. Freud took a deterministic view: biology and the psychosocial environment of the first 5 years of life are the determinants of the adult character. The existential position stresses the responsibility that the person has for his or her actions and affirms freedom of choice in each life (Yalom, 1980).

Existential ideas found some acceptance in North America with its ethic of self-reliance, autonomy and industry. There it combined with

From M.O. Aveline and B. Ratigan (1988) Interpersonal group therapy. In: M. Aveline and W. Dryden (Eds) *Group Therapy in Britain*. Open University Press, Milton Keynes, pp. 43–64.

* Written with Bernard Ratigan.

another German import – the future-directed, individual psychology of
Adler, as developed in the cultural theories of Karen Horney. Horney
was interested in the consequences for the individual of his behaviour,
and described characteristic patterns of relationships in which people
move towards, away and against or, more fruitfully, with others.

The interpersonal school of psychiatry began with Harry Stack Sullivan,
whose publications in the late 1940s located the concept of personality in
the interpersonal area. How we see ourselves is the summation of how
others have appraised us, he declared. Another strand – the ahistorical
element – was contributed by Kurt Lewin, a social psychologist and a
founder of vector psychology. People define themselves through the assumptions that they hold; when the same assumptions are held by others,
the field of forces so created restricts change. The training group
(T-group), an educative forum originated in the National Training Laboratories at Bethel, USA, in the 1940s–1950s, provided an environment for
change by bringing together groups of strangers who were encouraged
not to define themselves by a restatement of past roles, but rather to
explore the reality of their interaction within the T-group.

Many of the ideas that make up the interpersonal approach found
expression in the humanistic and later in the encounter movement that
swept North America in the 1960s and Britain in the early 1970s. Carl
Rogers was a spokesman for there being a potential for growth in each
person which could be released once a sufficiently facilitative psychological environment was created and perceived by that person. The
power differential between therapist and patient virtually disappeared as
the two met as equals in a true meeting, the encounter of the movement
that grew to meet the deficit of alienated modern life. In Martin Buber's
phrase, the healthy human relationship was 'I–Thou', not 'I–It'.

Formal small-group therapy in Britain has been powerfully influenced
by psychoanalytic object-relations ideas, and in particular those of splitting, projection and part-object. The notion of the group being moved
as a whole by unconscious shared processes provides a way of understanding the phenomenon of the group as a whole and of the individual
in the group; it complements the above described member-centred
focus on responsibility and encounter. The British writers Ezriel, Bion,
Foulkes, Whittaker and Lieberman have made their contributions,
some of which have become formalised in the group analytic school of
the Institute of Group Analysis in London.

The interpersonal approach is in common use in Britain but has little
formal recognition. Yalom, the Stanford psychotherapist, exemplifies
the key elements of the approach in his masterly textbook, now in its
third edition (Yalom, 1985). The approach shares some concepts with
group analysis, and is similarly concerned with improving personal
relationships. The interest in meaning and language when considering

the interpersonal acts of the group goes far beyond a behavioural analysis. Unlike the spectator role in gestalt therapy and psychodrama, the group is the vehicle for change, and its good functioning is given prime importance by the leader.

Underlying Assumptions

Theoretical underpinnings

Interpersonal group psychotherapy takes as its focus what happens between people – the actions, reactions and characteristic patterns of interaction that constrain the individual in his interpersonal life, and for which help in modifying is being sought in the group. A fundamental assertion of the approach is that each person constructs an individual inner world which is continuously being reconstructed through interactions with others, and which determines that person's view of him- or herself and others and affects what may be expected from others. A sufficiently secure assumptive world allows the validity of the model to be checked out and updated with significant others; a fear-ridden or rigid assumptive world leads that person to avoid or not attend to experiences which would suggest that revisions are necessary (Frank, 1974). The therapy group brings the individual face to face with how others are as people, and how inner assumptions powerfully determine the patterns of interaction that develop. That confrontation is fundamental to the process of change which lies dormant at the inception of an interpersonal group.

In contrast to psychodynamically derived group psychotherapies, the interpersonal approach emphasises five concepts explicated in existential philosophy and psychology: (1) human actions are not predetermined; freedom is part of the human condition; (2) the corollary of this is the importance of choice in human life and (3) taking responsibility for one's actions; (4) death is inevitable; but the nothingness of this can give meaning to life; (5) we are each engaged in a creative search for individual patterns that will give meaning to our existence. Writers such as Heidegger and Sartre have provided the philosophical and literary underpinnings for a psychology articulating these important, but often ignored, givens of human existence. Recognition of these by the leader gives a distinctive cast to the interpersonal group.

The existential concepts of responsibility, freedom and choice in interpersonal group therapy

Existential thought provides three important concepts for interpersonal group psychotherapy – responsibility, freedom and choice. Judged against the background of the dominant current Anglo-Saxon intellectual ideology of positivism, such concepts often appear dangerously woolly and more at home in left-bank cafés in Paris. They try to capture important ideas about human existence, which are difficult to quantify in the categories currently fashionable in scientific circles. Existential philosophy emphasises the significance for individuals of taking as much responsibility for or control of their own lives as possible; it is the obverse of the idea that people are victims of internal or external forces. It challenges the belief that biology, history, society, God or 'nerves' are the all-powerful determinants of a person's life. Thus, it is distinguishable from philosophical, psychological and sociological theories which see the human beings as objects rather than subjects, as recipients rather than as authors, to an important degree, of their own realities (Yalom, 1980). Reality, this approach suggests, is socially constructed (Berger and Luckmann, 1967).

The approach provides a clinical context where group members can move from being trapped in a personal world view in which they are passive victims of cruel circumstance, to a self-formed one where they can take more responsibility for their lives, relationships, symptoms and difficulties. The central therapeutic effect is not just an intellectual appreciation of an active world view but a lived experience in the group of enlarged freedom through experiences of new personal acts or refraining from maladaptive acts. This is not an absolute freedom but a tension towards a greater freedom and range of choices in human existence: a relative freedom within the context of a person's circumstances.

If the concepts of freedom and responsibility seem abstract, choice (the third concept), derived from existential thought, is more concrete. Human beings constantly exercise choice in their lives; their actions form their empirical reality, and reinforce value systems. However, the tendency of the human condition is not to want to shoulder responsibility for personal choice. In the group, members can come to see how, in that social microcosm, they are continually exercising choices which define their present being and predicate their future. For example, the very act of speaking or not can be seen as a simple example of the exercise of choice, rather than a given, immutable fact. The group can help show members the nature of their choices and identify characteristic, maladaptive interpersonal patterns; the group invites reflection on the desirability of the choices now made explicit and 'owned' by the individual, a process which prepares the ground for changing maladaptive choice patterns. From the microcosm of the group, the similar macrocosm of the member's personal and social worlds becomes clear. Hopefully, members will be able to exercise and experience responsibility and choice in the context of an extended sense of personal freedom.

The contribution of interpersonal theory

At the heart of interpersonal theory lies the concept of the self. William James' theory of the self makes an important distinction between the 'I' and the 'Me'. The 'I' is the pure ego of the individual while the 'Me' is the social self – that which is known to others. This was important for psychotherapy because it anticipated both role theory and object-relations theory. James (1890) believed that a person has as many social selves as there are individuals to recognise him and carry an image of him in their mind. The therapy group engages with and identifies the social self that a member offers. It encourages members to move into some of their other unexpressed selves and make them their own.

Lewin (1936) provided a useful analysis of the psychological space each person occupies. His field theory of vectors held that events are determined by forces acting on them in the immediate field rather than by forces at a distance.

The tenet that causation is a contemporary process has created some controversy in psychotherapy. Defending the importance of this, Ezriel (1956) argued that the unconscious structures the analyst uncovers in working with the patient are active in the present, and are not necessarily replicas of past realities and reactions. Interpersonal group therapy draws upon Lewin's concept of promoting change by 'unfreezing' the person from the restrictive assumptions that they have held and others in their social world have come to hold about them, by providing a new, unprejudiced psychological space for exploration, experiment, rehearsal and acquisition of new selves.

The third of the major figures in interpersonal theory was Harry Stack Sullivan (1953). His theory of interpersonal relations held that human experience consists of interactions or transactions between people. He held that an individual's history influences every moment of his life, because it provides a dynamic structure and definition of his experiences. Anxiety basically arises from threats to the individual's self-esteem; these threats are defended against by characteristic security operations. He took issue with Freud's idea that the basic structure of the personality was immutably laid down during the earliest years of life, and argued for a period ending at adulthood, depending on the sociocultural conditions, and partly on the idiosyncracies of each person.

His theorem of reciprocal emotion states that integration in an interpersonal situation is a reciprocal process in which (1) complementary needs are resolved or aggravated; (2) reciprocal patterns of activity are developed or disintegrated; and (3) foresight or satisfaction, or rebuff, of similar needs is facilitated (Sullivan, 1953). These Delphic statements appear to mean that (1) each person encourages others into certain role relationships, and (2) relationships are strengthened when needs are met and disintegrate when they are not. The interpersonal group shows members how they are the architects of their interpersonal 'fate'. In Sullivan's view there are always more similarities rather than differences between people. Interpersonal group therapy seeks to show how individual sufferers may shed some of their pain and rejoin the mainstream. In this they are helped by one another and by the leader, who is a participant observer and never just a mirror of the group process.

The contribution of analytic concepts applied to the process of the group

When the members of a group come together they begin a journey. If it is to be successful they need to be able to talk about themselves, their feelings, fears and worries, and about the other people in the group. From the outset the group will take on some of the characteristics of an individual being. Just as individuals distort and avoid, so do groups. The fears and reactions held in common move the group as a whole and this is the group process. The leader needs to be able to see this process at work and show the group members what is happening. If the process can be turned to good account it will lead to greater openness and sharing.

We have found the formulation of Ezriel (1950), a Tavistock analyst, helpful. This formulation can be applied to individual as well as to group processes. The group takes up a *required relationship* with the leader (or with the members in our extension of Ezriel's work) which safeguards them from being in the *avoided relationship* for fear that that would provoke the *calamitous relationship*. A clinical example may make clear this complex concept.

After some weeks in a therapy group, a 25-year-old mental health professional began missing sessions and turning up late when he did attend. He was black, articulate and slightly physically handicapped. The leader noted that the atmosphere was tense when the man was present and relaxed in his absence. The group showed false friendliness with the man so as not to confront him with his behaviour (the required relationship). The leader confronted the group with what they collectively were doing. It became clear that the man's knowledge of group therapy, his blackness, his combative verbal style and his physical handicap all contributed to a sense of relief when he was absent. The group avoided facing the negative feelings about this man (the avoided relationship). As the leader persisted with the exploration of the group process aspects, some resolution was achieved; fears subsided that the group would disintegrate (the calamitous relationship) if the man was challenged and retaliated in anger, or if the group faced unwanted feelings of racial prejudice.

The analytic perspective also shows other ways in which unconscious processes enter into the happenings of the group (see next section).

Key concepts

In being themselves in the group, members demonstrate their characteristic maladaptive interpersonal patterns. How these patterns are handled is what determines whether or not the group experience is therapeutic. Many elements (concepts) contribute to the therapeutic whole. In the group, members have the opportunity to gain *insight* into how they function with regard to others.

To derive benefit the member needs to have an *openness to being moved*, both by the interactions with others and in himself in his personal and world view. It may well require more than verbal assent or protestations of openness for the member actually to be at this stage in life. It is necessary for the members to be able and willing to assume *responsibility* for their own participation in the learning experience of the group. This means that they need to have a notion of themselves as agents, however minor, of their own destiny and not merely passive victims of biological, historical, social, religious or family forces. The experience of being in the group will help the member reveal his or her *assumptive world* (Frank, 1974), the accumulated set of inherited and acquired ways of looking at the world which profoundly affects a person's behaviour and relationships with other human beings.

In the group, members do not merely talk about their difficulties, they demonstrate them. Attending to the *here-and-now* interactions within the session is a characteristic feature of interpersonal groups. Members often find this focus difficult to cope with initially. What is experienced by the group in the shared present has an immediacy and accessibility which has a powerful potential to be therapeutic and is often frightening. It is a demonstration of the interpersonal difficulties and the start of a way forward towards the resolution of these difficulties. The ahistorical emphasis is dominant, and although, as in other forms of group therapy, the exploration of the origin of difficulties does take place, it is not necessary for change.

The major exchanges and activities within the group are disclosure, feedback, acceptance and risk taking. Disclosures are of two main types: 'secrets' from the past and the present outside the group which the discloser judges to be determining his or her behaviour and, secondly, information about the feelings being experienced in the here and now. The *Johari window* provides a facilitative model (Luft, 1966) (Figure 7.1).

Disclosure dismantles the façade that each presents to the other. The act of disclosing is almost universally accompanied by the release of emotional tension and the sense of a burden being lifted, unless the disclosure generates an attack. Feedback illuminates blind spots, aspects

Figure 7.1 The Johari window

	Known to self	Not known to self
Known to other	Public arena	Blind spots
Not known to other	Façade	Unknown

of the self that are obvious to others but not known to the self. In the process of feedback information is transferred between members, with the emphasis on accuracy and ownership. The person giving the feedback is encouraged to acknowledge that it is his or her own experience, and not claim universal authority for it, or exaggerate. Although many group members say that they are keen to receive feedback, they often find it hard to hear. It is particularly helpful in the resolution of oedipal difficulties, when the maturing person needs to be able to challenge authority figures, if members are able to give feedback to the leaders when they stand in that role in the transference. The concept of feedback is linked to that of acceptance. Feedback can be offered by one person to another: it need not be accepted. For it to be accepted, the timing has to be right and the recipient open and ready to hear. Feedback promotes the integration of buried parts of the self which have had to remain out of consciousness for fear of hurt or ridicule.

Underlying being able to use the group is the notion of risk, in that members have to put themselves to a greater or lesser degree in an exposed position. This may be just by being physically present but, if they are to derive maximum benefit, they have to take the risk of acting and especially of acting differently. This engagement will reveal the distortions that have brought the member to seek help through the exchange of group therapy.

Process refers to those unconscious elements which move the individual and affect the group as a whole. Individuals may, through the mechanism of *projection*, put into other group members and the leader archaic or otherwise inappropriate feelings and attitudes not fully based upon current experience. Likewise, in the process of *mirroring*, the member will have strong emotions about aspects of another's behaviour, words or actions which in fact represent aspects of his or her own personality. Often projection and mirroring are accompanied by *splitting,* which simplifies the complexity of human experience into two categories of good and bad. Similarly, the process of *scapegoating*, when the group blames a member for particular ills and tries to get rid of that person, suggests that the same hated aspects were present in other group members and being avoided. Parataxic distortions, the individual's proclivity to distort his perception of others, also provide valuable material which go to make up the work of the group. At times, the group will form a collective whole whose patterns make sense, once the required, avoided and calamitous relationships are identified (Ezriel, 1952).

As the group develops over time, a certain ritual dramatic quality will emerge out of the regularity of time and place. It will soon develop a life and personality of its own. The mood will vary between sessions but a culture of shared norms, expectations and values will emerge. Group cohesiveness will develop, through which members will, to a greater or lesser degree, come to feel that they belong, and this sets the stage for interpersonal learning (Bloch and Crouch, 1985; Yalom, 1985). A sense of group solidarity will be experienced which will counteract the feelings of alienation, isolation, individualism and fragmentation which the members will have hitherto experienced. One important component of this process is the sense of being of assistance to others in the group; this process is a vital element of the interpersonal group. Often members will report that what helped them in the group was not the contributions of the leader, however well intentioned, but the realisation of all being in the same boat, and that they had something to give to another human being. A sense of *koinonia* or fellowship will emerge.

There comes for each person in a group special moments when something has to be said or done. One of the Greek words for time, *Kairos*, expresses better than our English word how this is the right or acceptable moment (Kelman, 1969). This is linked with the concept of *catharsis,* which means the expression of strong emotion associated with stressful situations or memories.

The group can provide a *corrective emotional experience* in which earlier damage to a person can be worked through and, to some extent, repaired (Alexander and French, 1946; Frank, 1974). It provides a safe place where the *reflective loop* of doing, then looking back on what was done and understanding it, can be repeatedly entered upon. Finally, the group can provide a framework for individuals to grapple with finding *meaning* in their own existence and difficulties.

Practice

Change requires courage. A person joining and staying in a group gives up temporarily, and perhaps abandons altogether, the notion that he or she is self-sufficient and does not need help. Coming to terms with these losses is often difficult (Wolff, 1977); by temporarily giving up the idea that they are coping, the stage is set for work in the group which will enable them to develop a more realistic and solidly based life. Groups are threatening; they evoke all kinds of fears and fantasies. In the group, members do not just talk about their difficulties but demonstrate them to the other group members, to the leader and, eventually, to themselves. The member is asked to do that which is most difficult, and to say those things which cause them so much pain.

Generally, in a group meeting weekly for 1½ hours, it takes weeks or months for members to learn how to engage productively with the group. Significant personal change usually becomes apparent after 9–15 months' membership.

The goals of the group

The goal of the group is to create a temporary social world in which therapeutic learning can take place. Each individual has his or her own goal of resolving certain recurrent interpersonal difficulties. The leader has the goal of supporting the group and enabling the members to change, and the group members act as facilitators of that change; the leader fosters a climate in which enactments of interpersonal difficulties happen, and helps the group and individuals to identify what is happening.

The leader has the goal of identifying when the member or group is ready for work and needs to be able to create sufficient tension to bring the person or the group to the point of readiness for work so that insight and change can occur, while knowing that there is a narrow divide between risking too much and not risking enough. At the outset the leader must be willing to make a judgement that, with help, the potential member will, in time, be able to make use of the group.

Inclusion and exclusion factors

It is only necessary that potential members be able to understand and withstand the group process, and that they are able, perhaps with some help, to construe their difficulties in interpersonal terms. This means that they have recurrent difficulties in their patterns of relationships which are not purely intrapsychic and are potentially observable phenomena.

Those who should be excluded are the brain-damaged, the fragile, those who are not yet ready for a group and need the intimacy of the one-to-one therapeutic relationship first, and those who somatise completely. Additionally, those who deny the psychological basis of their difficulties are not good candidates for group membership. Those who recognise the role of the psychological but who waver in their recognition may be included, provided that they do not comprise the majority of the group.

The role of the leader

Selection and preparation

Careful selection and preparation help to make successful groups. It is important that, as far as possible, all members receive the same information and preparation for group membership. Boundary matters such as time, length, frequency of sessions, breaks and vacations are thoroughly rehearsed with each potential member. Commitment to the work of the group is important and questions of attendance and punctuality can be usefully discussed in the preparation session(s). The risk of drop-out may be reduced by anticipating with each member the interpersonal situations that may be specifically difficult for them; these often include intimacy, disclosure and the expression of strong feelings. If autonomy is a problem for a member, it is perhaps wise to insist that they come to the sessions under their own steam. Likewise, the all-important question of confidentiality needs discussion. The usual rule of no contact outside the group, and it is to be reported if it does happen, should be mentioned.

Many potential members have only a very vague idea as to what constitutes 'work' in the group. Careful checking with potential members will reveal what they think the group is for. It always pays to explain the ground rules of expressing what is being felt, especially if it is difficult to do so, and attending even when reluctant, and acknowledging this to the group. These injunctions are simple to state but, of course, touch on the heart of learning in a group. It is especially important to keep clarifying the potential members' unrealistic expectations because of the strangeness of group therapy for most people: for many, groups equal sociability, and therapy means being told what is wrong with one and what the solutions are.

It is useful to send a written statement of what is on offer when a place in the group is offered. This acts as a tangible record of the orientation session and can be a useful checklist for the member of what his or her responsibilities are (Bloch, 1979).

In an ongoing group the leader may choose to let a member, once accepted and thoroughly prepared, meet with volunteer group members before joining, and have a few recent group reports if available to help them orientate themselves.

The work of the leader

An important function of the leader is to identify the particular conflicts that are most likely to cause difficulties with group members and to construct a balanced group. Ideally, the group should contain members with a heterogeneous range of personality styles and a more or less

homogeneous level of interpersonal functioning. A variety of personalities is important because otherwise reinforcement of maladaptive
personal styles may occur, such as schizoid avoidance of intimacy, and
a group culture can develop which is antipathetic to change. Sometimes a change of membership may be necessary to break the collusive
maladaptive culture.

The leader as a facilitator of interpersonal transactions is neither
passive nor claims the centre stage, but will be both observer and
reflector of what is going on in the group. This latter role obviously has
echoes of the psychoanalytic perspective. The leader also models helpful group behaviour to the members, and in this the perspective is
linked with social learning theory (Bandura, 1971, 1977). In the interpersonal group, there is a special emphasis on language (see below)
with members being encouraged to speak for themselves and in the
first person. The leader models respectful attention, giving full weight
to what is being disclosed.

Technique

The beginning phase of the group is the most active time for the leader;
he has to maintain the group and encourage it to develop helpful
norms. If that work is done well, the leader can fade increasingly into a
background role leaving the active work to group members. His role
continues as an observer and a model of openness to learning, as
boundary setter and the person who may have to bring difficult topics
into the open. Prompting the group to look at the significance of breaks
and endings will almost certainly fall to the leader in the first instance.

In interpersonal group therapy, the major functions of the leader are to:

(1)   establish and sustain the group boundaries (selection and prepara-
      tion of members, the group room, receiving apologies, etc.);
(2)   model and maintain a therapeutic group culture;
(3)   provide an understanding of the events of the session;
(4)   note and reward member gains;
(5)   encourage members to take responsibility for their actions;
(6)   predict (and possibly prevent) undesirable developments;
(7)   involve silent members;
(8)   increase cohesiveness (by underlying similarities and caring in the
      group);
(9)   provide hope for members (it helps members to realise that the
      group is an orderly process and that the leader has some coherent
      sense of the group's long-term development).

One distinctive elective way of supplementing these functions is by
sending a written group summary to all members after each meeting
(Yalom, Brown and Bloch, 1975). The summary, a personal non-

authoritative account by the leader, gives a second opportunity to live the session and enhances its therapeutic impact; group norms are further shaped, and it is possible for the leader to add afterthoughts or highlight change. Finally the summary fills the gaps for the absent member.

When summaries are used, they are as much a part of the dynamic processes of the group as are the sessions themselves, as this vignette illustrates. In a training group the leader omitted the name of one member from the seating plan in the summary of the sixth session. In the next session, no mention was made of the omission but the omitted person seemed distressed and annoyed and was not participating actively. Finally, one of the members asked him what was the matter. He replied with a torrent of abuse directed at the leader and then subsided into tears as he told the group of his incredulity on receiving the summary and finding himself omitted. During the ensuing days he had tried to pretend to himself that it did not matter but he became depressed and agitated at the thought of attending the next session. Throughout his life he had doubts about whether or not he mattered to people. He had seen the leader as a good figure until the omission, which he had experienced as an annihilation. During the remainder of the session, he was able to set about working on his feelings of isolation, and this resonated with other members who talked about their own fears of being 'destroyed'. For many sessions afterwards members were preoccupied with the annihilation theme. Most of the group also admitted that on receiving the written summary they always anxiously scanned it for reference to themselves. The leader should note how members react to the summaries because this illustrates their interpersonal sensitivities (see Chapter 14).

Co-leadership

It is always more useful to have two leaders, preferably of differing genders. Besides providing support for each other, two leaders can adopt varying degrees of involvement and detachment; for example, if one leader is under attack by the group, the co-leader can help the group to examine what they are doing. Having a man and a woman leader often stimulates the exploration of sexual and parental conflicts.

Language, responsibility and group membership

The existential heritage of interpersonal group therapy places great emphasis on members being helped to take responsibility for their own lives.

As in all forms of therapy, close attention to the language group members use when speaking about themselves and others can be a productive source of material for the therapist. The words used can reveal, at first hand, how members see themselves and their position in the world. Often, they will speak about themselves as 'you', perhaps finding it difficult to say 'I'. This can lead to difficulties in trying to understand what they are talking about but, more importantly, may indicate an attempt to distance themselves from the emotional reality of their situation. To speak in the first person is to own one's experience. The leader encourages this, not as a rule but as a facilitative group norm. Indeed, the ability increasingly to speak for him- or herself, and an increase in clarity of a group member's language, are good indices of movement towards health and positive change. The ego or sense of self is being strengthened, and this is demonstrated through the words used to describe the self.

Microanalysis of the language of group members can reveal how they approach the question of taking responsibility for their own actions. Phrases such as 'You have to, don't you?' or 'You don't have any choice, do you?' signify an evasion of responsibility or a self-justification for seeing themselves as passive actors in their life (Schafer, 1983). By the gentle, persistent noting of such language the leader can encourage, first, an increased awareness and, secondly, an atmosphere in which members can begin to take responsibility and 'own' their behaviour and feelings through their language. The sequence might go as follows:

> You have to, don't you?
> I have to, don't I?
> I have to!
> I choose to.
> I choose not to.

Similarly, it is important for members to speak concretely about themselves and their experiences. Often the pronoun 'it' is used in such a way that the listener is left unclear about the speaker's meaning. Getting the group member to spell out exactly what 'it' is, is a basic interpersonal technique. The pronouns become nouns and the speaker is not only understood more clearly but comes to understand him- or herself better.

People come to therapy dissatisfied with the person they are, and feeling that in some sense, however tenuous, they have a different person within them that they could possibly become. In the group they can actually begin to speak about and, in so doing, articulate the kind of person they want to be, or the kind of things they want to do.

All the communications, both spoken and unspoken, are the subject of enquiry in the group. The meaning of the interactions that occur need to be decoded into what they say about how the person is and how they see themselves. The leader attends to gesture, movement and posture, as well as to the words spoken. The flow between members is another text to be understood – the kindnesses shown, the rage worked through, the ganging up and the acceptance.

The role of group members

Being in a group helps reduce isolation. Those seeking psycho-therapeutic help commonly believe that their misery and suffering are unique. Of course, to the solipsist, they are. Although not denying that an individual's experience is unique, his shared experience within the group powerfully demonstrates to members that they are not alone in their pain, and that pain and suffering are part of the human condition. In this way groups stand against much in contemporary Western culture which plays down suffering or marginalises it as individual weakness. By speaking of their own pain and hurt in the group, the members encourage each other to share and, temporarily at least, help carry one another's burdens. The 'telling' also helps put the individual's suffering into some kind of context. Much pain and suffering are endured in our society because of the fear of loss of face, and for the want of someone trustworthy to talk to. The group invites self-disclosure.

The group fosters tolerance. The leader can model this to those for whom it is a foreign language. In the early stages of the group, it is hard for members to understand that unconscious processes operate within the sessions and as such are part of the field of enquiry in the context of the exchanges. In their unconscious processes, both the individual and the group participate. For example, in projection, unacceptable parts of the self are discovered and put into others. Often in the process of mirroring, the member will attack this part of himself in the other before, usually with the help of the leader or another group member, coming to recognise that this is something for him to consider in himself. Similarly, the group may want to get rid of part of themselves, for example anger, by scapegoating this quality in a member who, to some degree, possesses it. Such magical actions need to be confronted by the leader.

Humour is important. To laugh is therapeutic and life is sometimes so dreadful and unfair that all that is left is laughter at the comedy of human existence. Laughter also helps counteract the dreadful gloom that can beset groups where all may be vying for the position of the saddest or most put-upon person (Bloch et al., 1983). Laughter with someone rather than at them, and laughter that comes out of shared experience is helpful. The leader needs to identify laughter which is (a) defensive and indicates that work is being avoided or (b) demeaning, which suggests that someone in the group is being scapegoated.

For many group members one of the greatest benefits of being in a group is the simple pleasure of being together with others and feeling safe – perhaps for the first time in their lives – a truly corrective emotional experience (Alexander and French, 1946).

It is the task of group members to be physically present and emotionally available for the events of each session. By being there and willing to work, the solidarity of the group is built up. Presence is shown by being open to what is going on in the group, by being willing to speak of their own feelings and thoughts, especially in the here-and-now of the group. It is especially important to speak that which is most hard to say when it is experienced. Attendance is essential. A quorum is necessary to ensure that work can take place. Sometimes group members with a history of earlier damage and unreliable or inconsistent relationships (including so-called helping ones) will find it hard to attend regularly or be on time (and in so doing they will demonstrate their difficulties). When these matters are raised, earlier hurts can be remembered, explored and faced. It may be through feeling let down, hurt or perhaps relieved at an absence or latecomer that a group member can come to recognise parts of his or her own biography or present experience that can be worked at and through.

In a group focusing on the interpersonal dimension all group members become peer therapists; all must refine their powers of observation and release their potential to be more than they were. Disclosures and feedback advance that end. In helping others, the helper realises his or her own skills and capacity and, in so doing, builds a stronger sense of self. The power asymmetry of the leader–member relationship can be somewhat redressed. Each can take his or her turn at helping, being the leader or, in the Indian sense of guru, being the person another can learn from. In such a situation group members have to face losing their previous belief that they were helpless, hopeless or incompetent. To be told by a group member that what one said or did was helpful is much more potent than being given 'feedback' by a therapist 'paid to say nice things'. Over time a group member can gradually regain (or even learn for the first time) competence in the simple tasks of being.

Group development over time

The natural history of the interpersonal psychotherapy group has three stages: a beginning, a middle and an end. Different factors emerge as being important at different stages in the life of the group; for example, at the start and for many weeks, it is important for the group to build collaborative norms. It may well be necessary for individuals to hold back on what seem like very pressing, personal disclosures until a sufficiently safe atmosphere of trust has been built. Confrontations, similarly, are often a more productive feature of a mature group which has the resources to handle them creatively.

The beginning, characterised by both hope and fear, sees the establishment of a therapeutic alliance between individual members, and between them and the leaders. In this stage the members settle down, thrash around trying to make sense of the chaos they experience, and try and discover the 'rules' of the group. They also start to show each other and the leaders their difficulties. Much of the talk is of topics far removed from the here-and-now experiences of the group and, therefore, safe. The leader is at his most active in this phase.

By the time the transition to the middle section takes place the focus will be more, but not exclusively, on the here-and-now. This section is much concerned with *keeping* the focus on the transactions in the group. The focus will often slip away, but the group itself will soon know this and experience these deviations increasingly as 'not working'. The thrust of the work will be in clarifying the distortions, risking saying what seemed impossible to say at the outset, in trying out new ways of being, in realising that some things cannot be changed but can be accepted.

As the group comes to face its end, much important work remains to be done, but as with all human relationships the group must end. The leader will have kept the ending in focus. Members will face, to a degree, the universal questions of death, the inevitability of mortality, the many unresolved griefs in their lives, the fact that all ambitions can never be realised, and that of the hopes that they brought to the group only some can be achieved; they will recognise how far they have come and what the group, the members and the leaders have meant to them.

Out of the experience, strength and individual potential will have been mobilised. Members will go forward alone to try new paths, but carry with them the shared experience of having in an important way transcended their previous being and of having been more the person they sensed they could be. Thus, each ending is a new beginning.

Duration

Groups may be open or closed, but to obtain maximum benefit, the members should ideally meet for 1½ hours weekly for at least 9 months, and preferably for up to 18 months or more. In our experience, an average duration of 12 months seems necessary, especially for patient groups, in order to allow for the full range of interpersonal difficulties to emerge and be worked on with any degree of lasting benefit.

Mechanisms of change

Change takes place in an interpersonal group in two overlapping and alternating stages. In the first, the group members come to see themselves more fully. In the second, through a lived experience of being different within and without the group, they move towards the persons that they might be if they were less fearful and conflicted. Yalom (1985), in an experimental study of 20 patients with good outcome following interpersonal group therapy (mean duration 15 months, range 8–22 months), showed that they valued in particular the interest of others, the catharsis of voicing feelings, and the sense of belonging. Top of 60 rank-ordered statements came 'Discovering and accepting previously unknown parts of myself', 'Being able to say what was bothering me instead of holding it in', and 'Other members honestly telling me what they think of me'. Replica studies show that promoting interaction among group members is a key therapeutic factor (Rohrbaugh and Bartels, 1975; Marcowitz and Smith, 1983). The selected statements refer to what Yalom termed 'interpersonal learning' within the social microcosm of the group: interpersonal learning has two elements, input and output, and these correspond to feedback and disclosure in the Johari window, described on pp. 91–92.

The group provides a sustaining structure in which the individual can take risks – the risk of discovering the contradictory and hidden aspects of him- or herself, the risk of venturing into new ways of being.

Typical problems and their resolution

Three examples are given of members presenting their problematic interpersonal selves in the group, the difficulties that this creates for the group is illustrated and an indication is shown of how this may be resolved creatively by the group with the help of the leader.

A pattern of playing safe resolved by disclosure and risk-taking

John always arrived in the group room at the precise time of starting. As the end approached he frequently looked at his watch, which he had programmed to bleep at the moment of escape. When the other group members eventually tackled him about his time-keeping he denied that it was important. The observation was repeated in the following weeks. Finally, he blurted out that he did not want anything to do with the other group members, who were clearly sick or they would not be in the group, and anyway he did not have time to spend on inconsequential talk. Another member pointed out that she had seen him walking round the perimeter of the building before the starting time looking very tense. John immediately denied this. The quiet disclosure of another group member of her fears of coming, of her sleeplessness the night before and of being seen coming into the building opened the way for John to tell the group that he was always frightened of arriving early because he did not know whether or not the leader would be present, and he was terrified of what the other members might get up to and say without the leader being present. So it was safer to arrive spot on time.

Recognising and then exploring the significance of the simple act of arriving on time initiated change. In the months that followed John began to recognise that he had the potential to risk arriving early and 'just chat and mess about'. He did not need the protection of the adult/parent/leader. He linked his clock-watching to the agonised days he used to spend in anticipation of his father's promised, but usually cancelled, visits, and to the hopelessness and self-hatred he subsequently experienced. *This had many resonances for other group members.*

John became a valued cornerstone of the group. His interpersonal interactions became much freer, and outside the group his relationship with his father became more equal. He experienced a new freedom to express himself with peers and authority figures, which was the antithesis of his previous fearful assumption that safety lay in never stepping out of line.

Self-hate hidden by inconsequential chat and resolved by peer-acceptance

Jean began most sessions by inconsequentially talking about matters outside the group. She usually had a tearful look about her but her wall of words usually stopped any interventions by either the group members or the leader. At first, the members of the group followed her lead and took the opportunity to engage in similar talk. The result was always the same: the chat went on and on and ended in that embarrassed silence that indicated that the group was not working. Gradually, the members of the group pointed out the pattern she initiated (and with which they colluded).

As the group progressed, Jean's chattering became less, though it never ceased completely. She gradually learned that the group members did care about her but she always remained cynical about the motives of the leader. The group helped by allowing her to display her difficulties. The endless chattering hid the tears. The tears were for her feelings of profound hopelessness and lack of self-worth. She felt that she deserved nothing, but she had begun to learn how to make a relationship both with the group and her boyfriend. She was able to make a world that fitted her better.

Rejection invited but averted by the action of the leader

Nicholas looked much older than his age suggested, and dressed in ill-fitting, too-elderly clothes. In his life, he felt he was an outcast. His family's professional standard of living, his nationality and his religion were at variance with the context in which he grew up.

In the group he adopted a stand-offish, cynical attitude. His physical posture betrayed a withdrawn avoidance: no eye contact, arms folded, usually leaning back. What comments he did make were hostile and dismissive of others' difficulties. He gradually became very isolated and somewhat the object of other group members' fear and dislike. The group began to resemble the world he feared and was, perhaps, instrumental in creating it. As the group developed he stood still.

After about 6 months, a member of the group quietly asked him why he had joined and why he kept attending, as he seemed not to contribute very much. Nicholas was hardly able to speak as a torrent of highly critical feedback came forth from many of the other group members. The leader felt that it was very important to protect him from the primitive and destructive forces in operation at this juncture, while preserving the importance of giving feedback. The leader encouraged the group to share with Nicholas how his behaviour affected them. He was also loudly told how much he was admired for still coming to the sessions in spite of his obvious discomfort. This illustrates the importance of members speaking for themselves, not assuming what is in the other's mind, and represents an important group norm for members.

Over the following sessions Nicholas was able to begin telling his story of how he had become such a brittle cynical person. He spoke of how he had acquired his defensiveness because he always felt an outsider and was frightened of opening his mouth lest his accent betray him. The family itself had developed a culture of silence, in which none of the members ever discussed the difficulties they experienced in living. Nicholas can be seen as an example of how a person's assumptive world was formed and maintained, and the quite powerful counter-experience needed to alter it.

Limitations of the approach

The chief limitation of the interpersonal approach to group psychotherapy is that it does not provide much space for individual exploration of severe psychological trauma. Although interpersonal group therapy emphasises the power of the group as an agent of change and healing, it does require that members are developmentally ready for the experience. This means, therefore, that it is inappropriate for those who are overly frightened of social settings and have not reached the psychological stage of seeing that other people exist as whole persons and not just as part-objects. Thus the narcissistic person, or those who can only relate to part-objects, will find it very hard to engage usefully in the group.

Similarly, the person who wants or needs a technological, structural method, such as is found in behavioural group therapies like social skills and assertiveness training, will not find the interpersonal approach appropriate. Neither will those who want to engage in an extensive exploration of themselves: they would find person-centred or analytic groups or individual therapy more useful. Whilst references to early life inevitably occur in any kind of group, the focus in the interpersonal approach is more on the here-and-now of current functioning than on the understanding of infancy and childhood. It is fundamentally ahistorical.

There is no neat matching of group therapy treatments to the variety of human problems. A more useful way is to see them as addressing different aspects of personal functioning. It is the purpose of the interpersonal approach to focus on helping members live differently with others; this is its priority.

Typical qualities of effective leaders

In contrast with more analytic ways of working, in the interpersonal approach the effective leader occupies a more involved position – but not so much as in leader-centred modalities such as gestalt, psychodrama and behavioural groups. Clearly, effective leaders need to be able to observe and give feedback, comment in a professional way on the group processes and their own part in them but, perhaps more importantly, they need to be able to model the qualities of effective group membership. These can be summarised as openness, willingness to change, to take risks and to be relatively undefended. The effective leader has, in addition, a belief that others can change and that, furthermore, this change comes about through the collaborative effort of members and leaders.

The effective leader does not believe that all the potency for change lies within him- or herself, but can see the potential of and in the group for effecting change. He or she can be comfortable with the leadership role changing, perhaps quite dramatically and almost, but never completely, withering away. Although the role might start off rather formally, it will soften as the group matures; this can usually be noted in the way the leader moves from being called Dr Y or Ms Z, to first names, rather like a good parent will be able to adjust to his or her offspring moving from childhood through adolescence to adulthood.

Finally, the effective leader is not unbending in his or her approach, but recognises that both he or she and the other group members are, as is often said, 'all in the same boat'. To take the maritime metaphor a little further, the leader is rather like the skipper of a yacht which would not be going very far without the crew, who in turn needs a skilled and experienced captain.

References

ALEXANDER, F. AND FRENCH, T. (1946). *Psychoanalytic Therapy: Principles and Applications*. New York: Ronald Press.

BANDURA, A. (1971). Psychotherapy based upon modeling principles. In: A.E. Bergin and S.L. Garfield (Eds), *Handbook of Psychotherapy and Behavior Change*. New York: John Wiley.

BANDURA, A. (1977). *Social Learning Theory*. Englewood Cliffs, NJ: Prentice-Hall.

BERGER, P.L. and LUCKMANN, T. (1967). *The Social Construction of Knowledge: A Treatise in the Sociology of Knowledge*. London: Allen Lane.

BLOCH, S. (1979). Assessment of patients for psychotherapy. *British Journal of Psychiatry* **135**, 193–208.

BLOCH, S. and CROUCH, E. (1985). *Therapeutic Factors in Group Psychotherapy*. Oxford: Oxford University Press.

BLOCH, S., BROWNING, S. and MCGRATH, G. (1983). Humour in group psychotherapy. *British Journal of Medical Psychology* **56**, 89–97.

EZRIEL, H. (1950). A psychoanalytic approach to group treatment. *British Journal of Medical Psychology* **23**, 57–74.

EZRIEL, H. (1952). Notes on psychoanalytic group therapy: II. Interpretation and research. *Psychiatry* **15**, 119–126.

EZRIEL, H. (1956). Experimentation within the psychotherapy session. *British Journal for the Philosophy of Science* **7**, 29–48.

FRANK, J.D. (1974). *Persuasion and Healing*, revised edn. New York: Schocken Books.

JAMES, W. (1890). *The Principles of Psychology*, 2 vols. New York: Holt.

KELMAN, H.C. (1969). Kairos: the auspicious moment. *American Journal of Psychoanalysis* **29**, 59–83.

LEWIN, K. (1936). *Principles of Topological Psychology*. New York: McGraw-Hill.

LUFT, J. (1966). *Group Processes: An Introduction to Group Dynamics*. Palo Alto, CA: National Press.

MARCOWITZ, R.J. and SMITH, J.E. (1983). Patients' perceptions of curative factors in short-term group psychotherapy. *International Journal of Group Psychotherapy* **33**, 21–39.

ROHRBAUGH, M. and BARTELS, B.D. (1975). Participants' perceptions of 'curative factors' in therapy and growth groups. *Small Group Behavior* **6**, 430–56.

SCHAFER, R. (1983). *The Analytic Attitude*. London: Hogarth Press.

SULLIVAN, H.S. (1953). *The Interpersonal Theory of Psychiatry*. London: W.W. Norton.

WOLFF, H.H. (1977). Loss: a central theme in psychotherapy. *British Journal of Medical Psychology* **50**, 11–19.

YALOM, I.D. (1980). *Existential Psychotherapy*. New York: Basic Books.

YALOM, I.D. (1985). *The Theory and Practice of Group Psychotherapy*, 3rd en. New York: Basic Books.

YALOM, I.D., BROWN, S. and BLOCH, S. (1975). The written summary as a group psychotherapy technique. *Archives of General Psychiatry* **32**, 605–613.

Chapter 8
The Practice of Group Psychotherapy with Adult Insulin-dependent Diabetics*

Introduction

Becoming ill and being ill are for most people major life changes that have to be coped with. For some, on balance, the experience may be positive in that personal and family resources are mobilised and the individual's determination, tolerance and understanding of others strengthened. For most, however, the experience is mainly negative, with major and repeated changes in body image, self-perception and social role being thrust on the individual, who frequently has to re-fashion his or her view of him- or herself. Likewise, others change and rechange their view of him or her. These alterations are partly functions of the nature of the illness, its stage, severity and treatment and, in part, of learned attitudes to illness in general and to the particular illness, both in the individual and those around.

Psychological problems have been emphasised as being common and a major factor in the course of diabetes in childhood (Tattersall, 1981) but it is often assumed that they are both less common and less important in adults with insulin-dependent diabetes mellitus (IDDM). What little has been written about the latter contradicts this assumption; Murawski et al. (1970) and Sanders et al. (1976) found that IDDM constituted a severe stress to many adult patients, and also to their families. Sanders et al. comment that 'anxiety and depression were most often related to fears for the future or worries about severe hypoglycaemia, which was described as the most frightening event in their life by 20%. In addition, early death and incapacitating complications haunted some patients, and the continuing regime of insulin injections,

From M.O. Aveline, D.K. McCulloch and R.B. Tattersall (1985) The practice of group psychotherapy with adult insulin-dependent diabeties. *Diabetic Medicine* 2, 275–282.

* Written with D.K. McCulloch and R.B. Tattersall.

regular meals, and constant vigil by patient or family weighed heavily on many, particularly those with no obsessive personality traits'. One possible way of dealing with such distress might be to bring patients together in groups to explore their problems, a technique which has an established place in medicine and psychiatry (Hadden, 1955), although its use in diabetes has been infrequent (Tattersall, McCulloch and Aveline, 1985). This paper describes two closed psychotherapy groups for patients with insulin-dependent diabetes. Quantitative analysis of the outcome in terms of diabetic control and psychological well-being have been reported elsewhere (D.K. McCulloch, M.O. Aveline, K. Knowles and R.B. Tattersall, unpublished data) and the aim of this paper is to describe the content and dynamics of the groups for others who wish to use this form of treatment.

Organisation of Groups

Most physicians probably know little about group therapy and may dismiss it because of the wide variety of techniques which have been lumped together under this heading (Yalom, 1975). Group therapy as defined here does not mean merely giving lectures to groups of people, neither is it simply a way of saving time by circumventing the traditional confidential consultation between one doctor and one patient. To us, it implies the use of the group process to alleviate illness or distress (Ryle, 1976). The model we used was member-centred, with a here-and-now emphasis (Yalom, 1975). According to this model the main therapeutic benefit in groups is seen as arising from interactions in a cohesive group, with discussion focused on current events and problems. The type of group approach with which this should be contrasted is the psychoanalytically derived approach of Bion (1961), who saw the leader as being central and dominant, focused attention on group members' interaction with him, and interpreted unsatisfactory relationships in terms of historical events and childhood experiences. Our intention was not to tell patients what to do, but to let them see their problems sufficiently clearly to be able to deal with them themselves, a principle summarised by the epigram, 'you can't do it alone but you alone can do it'. Members in our groups could share personal experiences, be accepted and helped by their peers, and improve their self-esteem through assisting others. The role of the leaders was to facilitate these processes; in particular, leaders tried to avoid the customary position of medical authority. They accepted criticism and encouraged free expression of feelings. They tried to prevent the group avoiding its prime task by escaping into social chit-chat or a technical discussion of diabetes and its management, in which the leaders would once more take on the role of medical experts.

Each group was led by a physician, one with 13 and the other 7 years' experience in the care of diabetes. Both had attended a 12-week course to prepare therapists to be group leaders. This course included a personal group experience of twelve 90-minute sessions plus seminars on the theory of groups. One leader (RBT) had also led a pilot therapy group for patients with diabetes the previous year. After each session, the leader made notes which were used as the basis for weekly supervision with a consultant psychotherapist (MA).

Membership

We wrote to 197 patients with IDDM of more than 6 months' duration, inviting them to participate in an 11-week course of diabetic lectures combined with group psychotherapy (McCulloch, Aveline, Knowles and Tattersall, unpublished data). Forty-six (22%) were sufficiently interested to be randomised, of whom seventeen were allocated to two psychotherapy groups. The groups met weekly for eleven 90-minute sessions; before each therapy session, all patients attended a 1-hour seminar on aspects of day-to-day management of diabetes. This was followed by a sandwich supper for half an hour. Nineteen patients were randomly allocated to attend only the 1-hour seminar and nine were not subjected to any intervention and were followed as controls.

Of the 17 patients who were allocated to the psychotherapy groups, 3 dropped out at various stages (see below), the remaining 14 being 6 men and 8 women with an average age of 40 ($\pm$ s.e.m. 3.2) years and an average diabetes duration of 13.9 ($\pm$ s.e.m. 3.0) years. Compared to the control or lecture-only group, they did not differ significantly with respect to duration of diabetes or level of diabetic control at the beginning of the study. However, they were significantly older ($P < 0.05$) and contained more men.

Content of Group Sessions

Both groups followed the same course as a closed psychotherapy group of similar duration for patients with neurotic and adjustment problems. Initially, members (see Tables 8.1 and 8.2) were hesitant with each other and reluctant to let their defences slip. This was particularly true of those with a long duration of diabetes, who initially had a strong tendency to preserve the status quo. They defended the expertise of doctors and excellence of the clinics and wished to deny that there were any problems in having diabetes or, if any were mentioned, implied that they were best not spoken of. In this way they avoided examining the reality of having diabetes and their dependence on medical services. Had they maintained this position throughout the group, little progress would have been made but, fortunately, some disclosed

Table 8.1 DMcC's psychotherapy group for patients with insulin-dependent diabetes (11 sessions)

Case no.	Sex	Age	Vignette	Diabetes Duration (years)	Diabetes Attitude to	Attitude to family	Expectations of group	Major disclosure (Session no.)	Change	Outcome category*
1	F	39	Vivacious, plump. Two children. Affluent	6/12	Openly proud of her diabetes. Inexperienced in treatment	Very positive	Increased self-awareness, friendship and support	Sadness at having 'cold unfeeling' autistic son (9)	Even more confident that she will cope	1
2	F	42	Primary school teacher. Two children, 21 and 19. Six months previously husband left her to live with 19-year-old student	21	Accepted. Not a secret. Resents diabetes when life going badly; then punishes herself by letting diabetes get out of control	Positive	Mutual support, new ideas, new directions	Husband deserting her, wanting acknowledgement, not pity (2). Emptiness of present life, two suicide attempts – resentment of husband's happiness (9)	More positive. No longer wanting to punish herself with loss of diabetic control, though still feeling her diabetes is restrictive. Beginning to enjoy her freedom	1
3	M	31	Shy, slight, computer operator. Secretly wanted to be racing driver. Single, lives alone	26	Denied and resented. Blames it for failure in life. Resentment surfaced as poor control in adolescence and non-attendance at clinics	No support. Little contact	Technical discussions	None	Happier. Wished had said more. Learned how others coped. Note: could not face saying goodbye so did not attend final session	1
4	M	30	Quiet, phlegmatic. Married, two children	18	Concealed, not normal but would talk about it if pressed	Positive	No idea	None	Coping better but doesn't know why	2
5	M	48	Obsessional, reticent 'old stager'. Secondary impotence, retinopathy	36	False front bravado covering misery	Positive	Information, help others	Childhood rejection (5). Diabetes began aged 11, belted by parents for high blood sugar, attempted suicide aged 14, beaten again (8)	Distressed by his disclosures but, also, relieved	2

6	F	51	Needs to be able to help others. Dependent upon clinics. Over complimentary to medical profession. Has to conceal inner feelings	Central in her life. Very active in British Diabetic Association	Frightened. Hostile	Help doctors understand	Husband frightened of injections (2). No sex. Daughter-in-law neglectful of children (8)	No obvious change	3
7	F	42	Quiet, pessimistic nurse. Ambivalently dependent upon clinics	Loathes diabetes and clinics. At home tries to deny illness	Husband frightened. Hostile	Help doctors understand as a way of replacing clinics	Diabetes a 'taboo' word at home. Husband frightened of injections, gets children to ring doctor if she has hypos (disgrace of having hypos) (3), husband hostile (9)	More positive about diabetes. Distressed by her disclosures	3
8	F	22	Black psychology graduate	Unknown	Unknown	Unknown	None	Attended part of the first session and then left saying she hoped to return. Appeared to be intellectually curious but not emotionally committed to the group	4

* Outcome category
1 = Good outcome: conflicts raised and substantially worked through.
2 = Moderate outcome: conflicts raised and partially resolved.
3 = Poor outcome: conflicts raised but no resolution, or uninvolved and unchanged.
4 = Drop-outs.

Table 8.2 RT's psychotherapy group for patients with insulin-dependent diabetes (11 sessions)

Case no.	Sex	Age	Vignette	Duration (years)	Diabetes Attitude to	Attitude to family	Expectations of group	Major disclosure (Session no.)	Change	Outcome category*
9	F	45	Chic, articulate, middle class. Married with two children. Previous experience of transactional analysis groups	5	A defect. Barely concealed resentment of doctors and insufficient support but doesn't want to be treated as an invalid or 'china doll'	Husband negative	Boredom. Understand self better and impact of diabetes on family	Double defect, diabetes and polycythaemia. Inability of husband to cope with this physical imperfection (9)	Experience of friendliness. Able to talk more openly about diabetes and ask for what she wants in clinics	1
10	F	19	Stutters. Mousy. Low self-esteem. Engaged	3	Hates being diabetic and having to attend clinics	Father and prospective mother-in-law hostile. Father fears injections	Learn about diabetes and what diabetics feel	Father went cold on her at 16 when she developed diabetes (2). Worried over having children (4). Rejection by prospective mother-in-law – gives son tea, patient nothing (9)	Increased self-esteem. More assertive with family and fiancé. Less frightened of hypos. Reassured that authority figures, like case 12, have problems too	1
11	M	22	Engineer, married to nurse	1	Positive	Uninvolved	Help ourselves, reduce sense of aloneness	Wife having affair (10)	Less alone with his problems. Improved communication with wife, but, also, increased awareness of the difficulties ahead	2
12	F	65	Vivacious, chatty. Public official. Pushed hard to join group, including calling herself 'an honorary 45'	4	Diabetes wrecked her life and marriage. Covertly seeking comfort	Husband now cossets her and does not treat her as a proper woman	To educate self and doctors about diabetes	Horrible distortion of marriage when diabetes began, from sweethearts to carer and invalid (1). Shame of hypos, would have to give up work if had one there (3). Mastectomy 6 years ago (6). Half a woman. Unlovable, unloved, wanting	Disclosed most. Unhappiness to the front of her mind. Still in need of support but not fully recognising it	2

	Sex	Age							*
13	M	31	Bearded civil servant joined group on session 3	Outwardly matter of fact	Uninvolved	Talk freely about personal problems and the restrictions diabetics pose upon themselves	Sister is a nurse and should be well informed and supportive, but isn't (3, 4)	Positive, but always has coped well	2
14	M	48	Tall, macho salesman. Conceals feelings and deals with problems by activity. Competitive	A problem to be solved. Forces family and colleagues to recognise his diabetes and help him with injections. Doesn't want to be dependent	Accepting	Uncertain	Severe, unreported hypoglycaemia when driving. Seen as threat to job (5)	Less defended and coercive. Beginning to accept that sharing difficulties is helpful. More aware of his problems	2
15	F	42	Shapeless, lumpy housewife	Superficially matter of fact. Hidden ambivalence shown by idea that she wouldn't want her daughter to marry a diabetic	Unknown	None	Daughter pregnant and unmarried at 16. Partner supported her at home (6)	Unchanged. Always able to cope. Aware that she, like others, has difficulty in keeping sugar levels down	3
16	M	25	Articulate, married just before onset of diabetes	Unknown	Wife refuses to give injections	Unknown	Got to be better than perfect at work to be acceptable	Developed paranoid delusions. Dropped out (5)	4
17	F	22	Fat, cheerful. Married with one child. Pregnant	Unknown	Husband involved	Unknown	None	Left after session 4 because of miscarriage	4

* Outcome category

1 = Good outcome: conflicts raised and substantially worked through.

2 = Moderate outcome: conflicts raised and partially resolved.

3 = Poor outcome: conflicts raised but no resolution, or uninvolved and unchanged.

4 = Drop-outs.

discordant emotional issues which, once accepted by the others, led to further disclosure and to the feeling that the group was 'a safe place, where one could say anything'.

An early theme was that diabetes might damage personal relationships; in session 1 a woman in her early sixties (case 12) blamed diabetes for the failure of her marriage. This was followed in session 2 by a 19-year-old woman (case 10) saying that up to the age of 16 years when she developed diabetes, she had been the apple of her father's eye, after which he 'went cold' on her. The same theme was followed in session 3 with a discussion of how much families actually help with day-to-day treatment. It transpired that parents and spouses were often phobic of giving insulin injections (cases 7, 10, 16), which reinforced the patient's sense of being different and alienated. Another common fear, brought up early in the group, was of becoming hypoglycaemic in public which was perceived as shameful and embarrassing as well as a threat to one's job and driving capacity.

For the first five sessions diabetic problems were the main focus. Diabetes had an individual meaning for each person, depending on the inherent stability of the disease, the remoteness or otherwise of complications, the reaction of key figures in the past and present, and the amount of non-diabetic tragedy in their personal life. Diabetes was seen by most as a shameful state which could be terrifying, and was in some way a defect and weakness (cases 7, 9, 10, 12). One woman (case 7), a nurse, revealed that diabetes was so taboo in her family that mere mention of it caused her husband to sulk, and if she had a hypoglycaemic attack, her husband got the children to ring the doctor and would not involve himself. He resented her attending the group and would remark, as she left the house, 'there's that paralytic going to her spastic group'. Another woman (case 9), an articulate woman in her mid-forties, saw diabetes as a defect, a view which was shared and compounded by her husband who could not accept that she was not the 'perfect woman he had married'. This theme of being ashamed of one's illness found expression in two ways: most concealed their illness from work colleagues, fearing that they would be rejected or might even lose their job (case 9). By contrast, one man (case 14) forced his workmates to accept his diabetes by deliberately drawing attention to it. The other manifestation was to worry about their children developing diabetes, to recall the hostility of parents, their boyfriends or girlfriends in their own adolescence (case 10), and to express doubt about allowing their own children to marry a diabetic (case 15).

In later sessions, other personal problems emerged and it became clear that there were traumatic events in members' lives other than diabetes. One woman, a 42-year-old schoolteacher (case 2) had been deserted by her husband for a 19-year-old student 6 months previously.

Her life was empty and she had attempted suicide twice. Inwardly she resented her husband's new-found happiness and tended to take the anger out on herself by letting her diabetes get out of control, which she admitted was a form of self-punishment. With the group's help, she became more accepting and began to enjoy her freedom. Another woman (case 12) was so desperate to be valued as a person that she misrepresented her age as 'an honorary 45' to gain admission to the group. One man (case 11) brought to the group the fact that his wife was having an affair. One member saw herself as having a 'double defect' of polycythaemia and diabetes (case 9). Both she and another patient (case 12), who had had a mastectomy 6 years earlier, bitterly resented the way in which their illnesses had transformed their husbands from partners to carers who treated them as china dolls.

Diabetes may be one traua among many. A 48-year-old man (case 5) maintained a false front of bravado in early sessions. He then revealed that from the age of 5 when he had first felt rejected, he had developed a way of protecting himself by suppressing his feelings. His parents had punished him for nocturnal enuresis, which lasted until he was 16. In session 7 he walked out when sex was discussed and, on returning the next week, said that he was impotent and had been told it was due to diabetes and untreatable. He went on, however, to relate that he had always been afraid of sex and had suffered from premature ejaculation even as a young man. He recalled how angry his parents had been when he developed diabetes at the age of 11. They beat him and he had tried to gas himself at 14. The group was supportive but he felt ashamed by his disclosure, and worried that he had slackened his rein too much. The group had helped him get into difficult and important areas, but he was not sure he wanted to be there.

The groups provided a forum where expression of powerful feelings and the telling of sad stories that could not be expressed elsewhere was encouraged and, more importantly, accepted. As the group matured, members' acceptance of each other was based on knowledge rather than faith. Acceptance raised self-esteem and countered the non-acceptance that so many had experienced from key figures. Those who entered into the spirit of the group became more assertive in their outside lives and, despite the pain that was revealed, there was much warmth and laughter and for some the ending was a real loss.

Technical Considerations

Leading a psychotherapy group is a skilled task like conducting an orchestra; the conductor's job is to bring out the best in the players for which he needs to know the score, what each instrument can do, and how a melodious whole can be created from the parts.

A group is made up of individuals, but fears and reactions held in common move it as a whole. This is the group process. Unconsciously the group may avoid (for example, by discussing the merits of plastic syringes) exploring members' ambivalence over dependence or anger over rejection, although they know that this is the purpose of the session. What happens is not random but follows an understandable progression which the leader must be able to see. The group process may be positive and impel members towards greater sharing and support. Once members feel secure with one another, they may feel sufficiently secure to ventilate deeper feelings and worries.

Part of the task of the group is to learn to reflect on what has happened between members and to understand the process involved, both as it applies to the group and to the individual. This *reflective loop* of doing, then looking back on what was done and understanding it, may be initiated by the leader or, as the group matures, by its members. Integral to the group process is how one person's problems resonate with another's, which may lead, sometimes after a period of hesitation or avoidance, to further sharing. In *mirroring*, members see in others, and often attack, aspects of themselves without necessarily recognising that the target also exists in themselves. The leader's role is to help members take back what they see in others and work on it in themselves. Talking about someone is often a prelude to talking about the same things in oneself. Discussing things, as it were, at second-hand in other people, tests whether the group is likely to accept you if it is disclosed that you have a similar problem.

To illustrate how the group process unfolded, we describe in some detail the main events during the second session in one of the groups. The group process was shown by the interaction between 'old hands' and those with recently diagnosed diabetes. In the first session those with long-standing diabetes presented themselves as having come to terms with it and being stalwart supporters of doctors and medical services in general. This position was threatened by more recently diagnosed members who were overtly critical. The precarious nature of the adjustment of the 'old hands' was illustrated by Joan (case 6 – names have been altered) seeking reassurance from the leader after the session because she interpreted his quiet style as a leader (in contrast to his active and authoritative posture as a diabetes expert) to mean that he was disappointed with her.

In session 2, the leader avoided an authority role by asking the group to summarise for a new member what had happened the previous week. Joan modified her previous position of 'everything's rosy' and revealed that her husband was frightened of injections. This led Marjorie (case 7) to say that her husband was so opposed to illness in any form that even the word 'diabetes' could not be mentioned in her home (resonance leading to sharing). This brought a counter-reaction (resonance leading to avoidance): George (case 5) wanted to seal over his emotional mess and critically advised that Joan's husband should be brought to the clinic for a 'telling off'. It was not until later (session 8) that his need to both cover up and re-enact his parents' own critical attitude became understandable, when he described his own rejection and attempt to conceal his emotions as a child.

The leader stayed with the emotional theme and brought in Shirley (case 2), whose husband had left her for one of his students. She wanted her situation acknowledged but did not want pity. George said that members did not have to discuss their personal life in the group. He was both being self-protective towards Shirley (individual process) and speaking for the part of the group, which feared stirring up past and present hurts (group process). The next half hour was spent happily and unemotionally discussing which needles were best (group process leading to flight).

The leader gently confronted the group with what was happening. George, speaking for himself and the group, explained that he bolstered his inner doubt with a public mask of bravado, and admitted having done this (reflective loop). This honest undermining of shared defences brought a counter-reaction from Joan who wanted 'to keep the hatches on' and returned to praising doctors, saying that diabetics should not worry if they attended a good clinic (resonance leading to avoidance).

Each person will be vulnerable to varying degrees in his or her areas of *core conflict*. Normal developmental stages of trust, separation, assertion and sexuality may not have been mastered and will have left residues of conflict. Diabetes poses special problems when an aspect of it coincides with the core conflict. Conflict may either be described or enacted and, when this happens, the group can initiate change if it encourages the person to act differently and itself responds, so as to negate what for the person in question has become a demoralising, self-fulfilling prohecy about how others will react to him. This is called the *corrective emotional experience* (Alexander and French, 1946).

These two elements were illustrated in the ninth session of one group. Self-worth had emerged as a central theme and several members had voiced their feeling that they were seen as imperfect and might easily lose the acceptance of others. Mona, a hesitant 19 year old, whose core conflict centred on a fear of rejection if she was assertive and independent, described a typical interaction with her fiancé's mother; the latter had become hostile when Mona developed diabetes 3 years earlier, and carried this to such a length that, when Mona visited, the mother made tea for her son but not for the girl. Mona habitually dealt with her conflict by adopting a pleading and ultimately

demeaning posture. This group reduced her sense of self-critical isolation by sharing similar experiences and by being warmly supportive
(corrective emotional experience). Subsequently she worked out a
solution which was good for her but was neither all-out confrontation
nor avoidance. By the tenth session she reported a pleasing move
towards greater independence.

Outcome

Joining a psychotherapy group is like being on a big dipper; you may
want a ride but find the reality unpleasant. Once on it is hard to get off
before the end, and sometimes you hold your breath and wait for it to
finish. At best the experience is a shock, but nevertheless invigorating
because one's usual boundaries have been extended and one has
passed successfully with others through a trial. These different responses highlight the mixed experience of being in a group. It offers a
unique opportunity to put aside defences and learn through interaction
that what seems terrible when locked away inside loses its power
when shared, and that conflicts can be resolved and a more successful
adaptation made. However, for some the opportunity is a threat to the
adaptation and defences they have built up over the years – the familiar
is safe, the new dangerous.

The effectiveness of psychotherapy, either group or individual, has
been questioned, partly because of the way patients are selected, but
also because formal trials have rarely been carried out (Editorial, 1984).
The criticism is ill-founded, though the call for research is welcome
(Aveline, 1984). Patients in this study were randomly allocated to
therapy groups or lectures alone, but there is little doubt that those who
participated may be unrepresentative of insulin-dependent diabetics as a
whole; only a quarter of patients who were invited to participate accepted, and there is no way of knowing how many agreed to take part
because of particular personal problems with which they hoped to gain
help. In fact, most of the 14 patients who completed the group therapy
sessions had major personal problems in addition to diabetes.

Metabolic control and psychological outcome were assessed objec-
tively by means of haemoglobin A_1 and purpose-designed questionnaires 3 weeks and 9 months after the end of the groups, as described
elsewhere (McCulloch, Aveline, Knowles and Tattersall, unpublished
data). As compared to the lectures-only and cnntrol group, there were
no significant differences in either haemoglobin A_1 or measures of
adjustment to life in general or diabetes in particular. Another, more
subjective but equally valid, way of assessing the effect of these groups
is to grade patients into categories based on the use made by members
of the sessions. We have chosen four categories:

1. A good outcome, where conflicts were raised and substantially worked through.
2. A moderate outcome, where conflicts were raised and partly resolved.
3. A poor outcome where conflicts were raised but not resolved, or where patients remained uninvolved and unchanged.
4. Drop-outs.

Good

Five patients (cases 1, 2, 3, 9, 10) both raised conflicts and substantially worked through them. For example, a woman (case 2) who had been deserted by her husband came to terms with her loss and felt less resentful and oppressed, both by her desertion and by diabetes. She regained a sense of optimism and purpose. Case 10, a 19-year-old woman, was greatly helped by seeing that older authority figures had similar problems to her own. She became more assertive with her family and fiancé.

Moderate

Six patients (cases 4, 5, 11, 12, 13, 14) raised conflicts but only partially resolved them. Case 5, an obsessional 48-year-old man, had over many years developed a false aura of cheerfulness to cover his inner misery. The group helped him share problems, past and present, but there was too little time for him to consolidate this substantial shift. He felt exposed and at the end raised his barriers again. Case 14, a 'macho' 48-year-old salesman, made no major disclosures but did come to appreciate the value of sharing difficulties. Previously he had denied his problems and forced others to accept him as normal. A longer group might have helped him more.

Poor

Three patients (cases 6, 7, 15) either did not resolve their conflicts or remained uninvolved. Case 6, a 51-year-old woman, felt she had to conceal her inner feelings. Her husband was frightened of injections and hostile to her diabetes. They had no sexual life together and she coped by being dependent on her doctors, whom she idealised. Her expectation of the group was that she would help the doctors rather than herself. Her difficulties at home were raised but not resolved.

Drop-outs

One patient (case 8) was intellectually curious about, but not emotionally committed to, the group and dropped out after the first session. Two others dropped out later; one, case 16, a well-educated, articulate young man was married to a fervently religious black woman and had developed diabetes 8 months previously, just before his marriage. His wife refused to give injections, which was difficult for him to discuss as he felt he had to be perfect to be accepted. Half-way through the study he developed a psychotic illness, with religious overtones and paranoid delusions. The third drop-out (case 17) left because of a miscarriage after session 4 and never returned.

Overall, patients whose expectation of the group was that they would gain a greater understanding of themselves and reduce their sense of isolation did better than those who attended to learn more about diabetes or help the doctors. In comparison with other psychotherapy groups, the present one was relatively short and it may have been unrealistic to expect more positive results, in view of the fact that those participating had had diabetes for an average of 14 years, so that their maladaptive behaviour patterns were likely to have been relatively fixed. Against this, it is also possible that our clinical judgements of good or moderate outcome were inflated by end-of-group optimism and people being made bolder by the support of the group. We stress that the groups were not simply a forum for factual discussion, education or support. Much emotional pain was disclosed and worked through, leaving an overall impression that members welcomed the opportunity to 'get things off their chests' in a constructive atmosphere. Several gained in self-respect and self-confidence, whilst others were disturbed by what they had to face. For others, the work of the group was only the beginning of a re-evaluation which will take years to complete. Like the management of diabetes, which is a continuing process, psychotherapy has no clear starting and stopping point and loose ends are inevitable.

Guidelines for Leading Groups

Clearly the leader is not just a chairperson, but has to be ready to intervene when individual or group processes are subverting the best purpose of the group. The leader needs to maintain an optimum 'temperature' for psychological work. If it is not hot enough, the group loses creative tension. If it is too hot, people get frightened: the warning signs of this happening are restlessness and mounting agitation, which signal the possibility of someone walking out and not coming back. The leader must be fair and proper in his conduct. For example, to give a member a lift home (as was done by one of the present leaders) is kind, but smacks of favouritism; similarly, names and addresses of members are privileged information and must not be disclosed without permission.

The leader must avoid becoming the centre of attention. His job is to facilitate members talking to and helping each other. The diabetologist who decides to lead a group of diabetic patients is in a particularly difficult position; in his everyday work he is the centre of attention and authority in the clinic but, in the group, he must make clear that he is not there as an expert to answer technical questions. Preferably the group leader, if a diabetes specialist, should not have clinical responsibility for members of the group. Diabetic clinic staff are expert in their own field, but when leading a group, they must avoid being seduced into the role of expert, protector and patriarch. The leader should foster cohesion and acceptance by showing an interest in, and accepting, everything that happens in the group. He must be aware of emerging personal agendas, often signalled by trial disclosures or anecdotes about outsiders. The temptation to heal major problems in a short time should be resisted. Finally, he must ensure that the group starts and stops on time and abides by rules which are agreed by all members from the outset.

Conclusions

As far as we know, the use of group discussions in the management of diabetes began with, and has virtually been confined to, the work of Groen and Pelser in Holland (Pelser et al., 1979; Groen and Pelser, 1982). The stated purpose of their groups was 'to offer diabetic people the opportunity to meet to discuss under expert guidance the difficulties associated with their condition, as well as the general problems of life'. A major difference between their groups and ours was the duration of therapy; in the usual weekly psychotherapy groups, members take from 3 to 6 months to settle down and understand how the group can benefit them, and improvement in function only starts in the next 6 months. The Dutch groups met on a weekly basis for 48 weeks, and in this context our study of 11 weekly sessions was very short, although labour-intensive for the leaders who had to do it in addition to, rather than instead of, ordinary diabetic clinics. We feel that our diabetic groups had two advantages over ordinary psychotherapy groups: first, members had in common their illness, which accelerated the development of cohesion. Secondly, the limited time available concentrated minds and feelings and compressed into a relatively short time the sort of evolution that occurs in a longer group.

Does the leader need to be a doctor, expensive to train and pay? Our answer is a qualified 'yes'. Doctors are authoritative figures, and in illness like diabetes great expectations of help are placed on them. That dependency, with its corresponding loss of strength in the patient, saps initiative and self-confidence, qualities which are essential in an illness that demands unrelenting commitment to self-monitoring and self-treatment. Furthermore, the usual clinic visit discourages the expression of ambivalence and legitimate criticism by the patient. The group changes this relationship, and having a doctor as leader was an important factor, it being noticeable that members grew in authority as the group progressed and came to recognise its own expertise. A nurse practitioner or other skilled member of the clinical team would probably also make a good leader, but we feel that a specialist from another discipline, such as a psychotherapist or psychiatrist, would encourage splitting the emotional aspects of the patient's life from the physical, something medicine is all too ready to do. In the studies of Groen and Pelser (Pelser et al., 1979) patients were much less satisfied and the rate of default was higher when the group was led by a psychologist rather than by an internist.

There is clearly an overlap between what happened in our group and what happens in self-help groups such as local diabetic associations. Nevertheless, self-help groups are different in not being formally structured, not having such a self-reflective purpose, and in having leaders who act as chairmen rather than therapists. The interactions in our group were complex, and we would strongly urge anyone setting up a group to make sure they have the back-up of regular supervision by an expert in group therapy. It has been shown that untrained therapists, who tend to become more authoritarian as the groups progress, or leaders who are intrusive, demanding and aggressive, can make patients worse rather than better (Ebensole, Leiberman and Yalom, 1969; Lieberman, Yalom and Miles, 1973).

As with the Dutch studies (Peter et al., 1979; Groen and Pelser, 1982) discussion in our groups went far beyond the technical aspect of diabetes. It clearly met an unsatisfied need, although we must stress again that patients were to some extent self-selected. Nevertheless, we are sufficiently encouraged by the results to recommend further use of this approach with insulin-dependent diabetics, and feel that in future it might be profitable to vary the format by increasing the number of sessions, adding additional sessions at monthly intervals for a further 6 months, and selecting particular populations, for example, patients with newly diagnosed diabetes or those with specific problems, such as obesity, major complications, or those whose disease is difficult to control.

Acknowledgements

During the course of this work Dr D.K. McCulloch was supported by a grant from the British Diabetic Association.

References

ALEXANDER, F. and FRENCH, T.M. (1946). *Psychoanalytic Therapy: Principles and Application*. New York: Ronald Press.

AVELINE, M. (1984). What price psychiatry without psychotherapy? *The Lancet* 2, 856–859.

BION, W.R. (1961). *Experiences in Groups*. London: Tavistock Publications.

EBERSOLE, G.D., LEIBERMAN, P.H. and YALOM, I.D. (1969). Training the non-professional therapist. *Journal of Nervous and Mental Disease* 49, 385–392.

EDITORIAL (1984). Psychotherapy: effective treatment or expensive placebo? *The Lancet* 1, 83–84.

GROEN, J.J. and PELSER, H.E. (1982). Newer concepts of teaching, learning and education and their application to the patient–doctor cooperation in the treatment of diabetes mellitus. *Pediatric Adolescent Endocrinology* 10, 168–177.

HADDEN, S.B. (1955). Historic background of group psychotherapy. *International Journal of Group Psychotherapy* 5, 162–168.

LIEBERMAN, M.O., YALOM, I.D. and MILES, M.B. (1973). *Encounter Groups: First Facts*. New York: Basic Books.

MURAWSKI, B.J., CHAZAN, B.I., BALODIMOS, M.E. and RYAN, J.R. (1970). Personality patterns in patients with diabetes mellitus of long duration. *Diabetes* 19, 259–263.

PELSER, H.E., GROEN, J.J., STUYLING DE LANGE, M.J. and DIX, P.C. (1979). Experiences in group discussions with diabetic patients. *Psychotherapy and Psychosomatics* 32, 257–269.

RYLE, A. (1976). Group psychotherapy. *British Journal of Hospital Medicine* 19, 239–248.

SANDERS, K., MILLS, J., MARTIN, F.I.R. and HORNE, D.J.D. (1975). Emotional attitudes in adult insulin-dependent diabetics. *Journal of Psychosomatic Research* 19, 241–245.

TATTERSALL, R.B. (1981). Psychiatric aspects of diabetes – a physician's view. *British Journal of Psychiatry* 139, 485–493.

TATTERSALL, R.B., McCULLOCH, D.K. and AVELINE, M.O. (1985). Group therapy in the treatment of diabetics: a review. *Diabetes Care* 8, 180–188.

YALOM, I.D. (1975). *Theory and Practice of Group Psychotherapy*, 2nd edn. New York: Basic Books.

Chapter 9
Personal Themes from Training Groups for Health Care Professionals

We talked far into the night, as friends do when they meet again, amid the homely village smells.
'How long have you been hearing confessions?'
'About fifteen years . . .'
'What has confession taught you about men?'
'Oh, confession teaches nothing, you know, because when a priest goes into the confessional he becomes another person – grace and all that. And yet . . . First of all, people are much more unhappy than one thinks . . . and then . . .'
He raised his brawny countryman's arms in the starlit night:
'And then, the fundamental fact is that there is no such thing as a grown-up person . . .'

André Malraux (1967)

Health care professionals often feel unhappy and not grown up. Their work is stressful and their institution may either be unsupportive or their own conflicts may inhibit them from taking advantage of what support exists. This paper describes the personal themes presented in the training group component of an annual group psychotherapy course, and considers the implications for group leadership and the training and care of these workers.

The Group Psychotherapy Course

In 1976, the author devised an annual, introductory, multidisciplinary, group course which provides practical, systematic training for inexperienced leaders in 12 weekly sessions. Each week there is either a 1-hour seminar on theory or a practicum of leadership skills; after a sandwich supper the 20–30 participants divide into two or three 1½-hour

From M.O. Aveline (1986) Personal themes from training groups for health care professionals. *British Journal of Medical Psychology* 59, 325–335.

training groups, each with a single leader. Over the years it has become evident that, for the trainees, this group experience is the most valued component of the course.

The set readings for each week are based in the main upon the second edition of Yalom's (1970) textbook. Yalom provides an existential, interpersonal model which is readily applicable to the relatively unstructured therapy that most trainees practise in their work settings. The model stresses commitment, self-disclosure, spontaneity and openness to learning from interaction. The training groups follow this model and are formally intended to develop the sensitivity of members to the needs of others, to increase self-knowledge, and to deepen awareness of group process.

An innovative feature of the course has been the use of written reports as an aid to training (see Chapter 14). Briefly, in the first seven courses a detailed typewritten report, 1000–2000 words in length, was posted by the leader to members after each meeting. The content of the report interwove three elements: (1) a naturalistic narrative of the meeting; (2) the leader's view of the dynamics of both the group and individual members; and (3) an explanation of why the leader chose to intervene in a particular way, or not to intervene. In style, the reports emulated the form described by Yalom, Brown and Bloch (1975). In courses 8–10 in order to enlist the active participation of the trainees, a new format was introduced. A brief four-question structured report focusing on group themes and leadership skills was sent to members by the leader after each meeting. Before the report arrived, members completed their own structured reports about group themes, significant events and problems for the leader. Through the two reports, members have been able to compare their perspective with that of the leader. After the third and ninth meetings, members' reports were circulated to each other, thus providing many versions of the same event. In addition, after the sixth meeting, the leader sent to each member a confidential tentative evaluation of their potential as a group leader. Most members elected to discuss their evaluations in their groups. The personal themes reported in this paper have been derived from an analysis of the written reports and the post-course questionnaire.

Ten courses have been held; 210 health care professionals (75 men, 135 women), mainly employed in mental health, have taken the training. There have been 21 training groups and 6 leaders (one consultant and one senior registrar in psychotherapy, one consultant in general psychiatry and one in child guidance, and two counsellors from university services, all with extensive experience as group leaders). Psychiatrists in training are encouraged to take the course as an elective option in their second year, but more senior registrars than registrars have done this. In the beginning, psychiatrists and nurses constituted the

largest professional group, each contributing one-third of the membership. Subsequently, the proportion of doctors has declined, with social
workers, and especially occupational therapists, increasing their percentage. Overall, nurses are the largest group at 28 per cent, followed
by doctors at 22 per cent and social workers at 18 per cent; in these
groups 17, 11 and 31 per cent respectively have been senior members
of their profession who have attended to renew or develop new skills
and, in at least two cases, to restore their confidence in group therapy.
A welcome development has been the participation of physicians and a
specialist nurse in diabetes, which has led to a research study (see
Chapter 8). Occupational therapists have accounted for 13 per cent of
participants. Psychologists, counsellors and clergy, teachers and probation officers have each contributed around 6 per cent to the number.
The participation of two art therapists and one drama therapist in the
last two courses has marked the establishment of these two new professions in the National Health Service.

Process Development in the Training Groups

Within the brief period of 12 weekly meetings, the development of a
cohesive working group is possible. Three factors foster that development – the within-group focus, its composition, and the reinforcement
of the group experience by the seminars and written reports. Two
factors oppose – the limited time for working through conflicts, and
the ambivalence of some members about the task. The leader makes a
vital contribution but the effect greatly depends upon how members
and leader combine; a 'positive confrontation' style of leadership (Alexander, 1980) appears to be the most fruitful.

In these groups, 'storming' (the second stage in Tuckman's (1965)
developmental sequence: forming, storming, norming, performing) has
been the most crucial for the final outcome. For members, the choice
has been between staying defended or moving towards meeting in
dialogue. From the first course, a twofold anxiety was evident: members feared adversely affecting their careers by disclosing personal difficulties to colleagues from the same place of work, and to a lesser extent
they were loath to bring to the group work issues that might show their
institution in a poor light. In recognition of this, and in line with the
interpersonal model being taught, the focus of the group has been on
here-and-now interactions within the group, and external events only if
they are volunteered; the groups were thus not primarily institution-
centred. An advantage of the within-group focus is that it 'unfreezes'
the individual from the external social matrix (Lewin, 1947) and sets
the stage for potential change. The fact that the groups are closed
facilitates the rapid development of a cohesive atmosphere. In compos-

ing the groups, every effort was made to balance the sexes and separate those who work together.

Though these procedural devices partially relieve anxiety, the underlying fears have, of course, to be worked with in the group. Without exception, each group has been concerned with confidentiality and has needed to set limits on how much of the content of the meetings can be revealed to spouses and colleagues. Intimacy, both desired and feared, is the theme whose resolution has divided members into a minority for whom the end of the course is a welcome relief, and the majority for whom it is a significant loss.

Personal Themes from the Training Groups

Personal tragedy which cannot be expressed at work for fear of being thought weak

It will come as no surprise to anyone with experience of training groups, especially those held in the 'hothouse' of residential workshops, that much personal tragedy lies close beneath the surface of able, working health care professionals. The members of one group spent nearly every session in tears, and were preoccupied with loss both in the outside world and within the training group.

In another group one woman was helped to value herself and to assert herself appropriately. Key elements in her biography and circumstances had together eroded her confidence in herself as a mother and at work. A critical father whom she had, by turns, vainly tried to please and defy, a failed marriage and failing performance at work combined to reinforce her doubts about herself. In the group, members worked to undo the guilt she felt when sharing her difficulties, and the inhibition she had over expressing anger. In the post-course questionnaire, she reported that her expectation of her group was that 'it would be very threatening and disturbing, but I found myself able to direct my anger to the right source, and feel less guilty about things and more able to value myself as worthwhile'.

A similar conclusion was reached by a man who had been 'incarcerated' in hospital with a mysterious illness between the ages of 1 and 4. The separation from his parents had left a residue of uncertainty in their relationship. As the group became more intimate, his sorrow for that early loss surfaced. He was supported in his sadness. After the course had ended he wrote: 'I unexpectedly breached the inner wall around my feelings about being away from my parents in childhood. I felt more self-esteem as the result of this experience.'

The experience of tragedy and sadness in the life of the health care professional, and especially the mental health worker, provides valuable, and perhaps necessary, sensitisation to the harsh personal realities of our world. Storr (1979), writing about the personality of psychotherapists and their work in understanding other human beings, underlines the powerful therapeutic force of the therapist being 'unequivocally on the side of the patient'. He continues:

> Successful therapists generally possess an especial capacity for identifying with the insulted and the injured . . . Psychotherapists often have some personal knowledge of what it is to be insulted and injured, a kind of knowledge that they might rather be without, but which actually extends the range of their compassion.
>
> (Storr, 1979, p. 173)

Having personal problems to explore in the group is clearly a factor in prompting application for this course, but the frequency with which such experiences are disclosed, the value placed upon the degree of resolution possible in these brief groups, and the seeming absence of emotional support in the institutions where members work, point to an unmet need among staff. Members have often expressed their regret at the lack of supportive settings in which difficulties, past and present, could be explored and, furthermore, felt that their professional role was incompatible with such expression. To disclose personal problems was to invite the accusation of undesirable weakness from others, and from their rigid, internalised role model which stated that carers have to be strong (see below).

Despite the explicit aim of the course to teach the use of groups as a means of psychotherapeutic change, and the opportunity that the training groups offer for personal exploration, members have been ambivalent about this prospect. The common anxiety was expressed by one member, who expected that the group would be personally threatening, that his feelings would be almost overwhelming to him but trivial to others, and that the others would show themselves to be more integrated, warmer and insightful – in the event, his experience was the reverse of his anticipation. Some members have had a definite but undeclared wish that their group would fail to reach the stage of 'performing', that is, engaging in therapeutic work. If the group arrests at a superficial level, denied needs may not have to be faced and emotional exchanges may be avoided. Regrettably a few members, temperamentally unsuited to group work, have been directed by their superiors to take the course; the reward for them of the group failing is being spared working in groups in the future.

Sometimes the personal problems disclosed have been too extensive to be resolved in the group. Members who know their psychological nature have appreciated this and have set limits to what was to be explored and have gone to seek formal therapy either individually or in a group after the course has finished. The leader has needed to set limits for some, particularly those in whom a paranoid core is triggered by the growing intimacy in the group, and to confront ways of being in the group that are destructive to the individual and to the group. This management problem is considered in the discussion.

The helpless helper

Isolation within their own profession or in the institution is a common theme. Colleagues at work have been seen as not comprehending the psychotherapeutic principles advocated by the member, or promoting treatment programmes that run counter to those principles. The institution has been seen as distant and inhibiting to individual creativity, or ready to squash initiatives that challenge the status quo. One nurse was sure she would be sent to a backwater, a long-stay ward, if she voiced her criticisms.

From the point of view of the leader, the temptation is to collude with the defensive mechanisms of splitting, in which the group members are seen as 'good' and the institution as 'bad', and thereby secure greater group cohesion. The price of not interpreting the projective base for *some* of these perceptions is a perpetuation of an unreal 'us' and 'them', good and bad polarity which excludes examining the doubts, uncertainties and problems of those whose work it is to care for others (see below). When the external situation is held to blame for the failure of treatment, the doubts of members about the effectiveness of their own treatments are stilled. At a deeper level, there is the frustration experienced by members in working with patients whose internal world is so persecutory that no image of the therapist as a basically helpful person can be maintained, and whose devaluation of the therapist renders him or her hopeless and helpless (Adler, 1972). The frustration is displaced outwards. Nevertheless, the frequency with which isolation is expressed, and the readily apparent sustenance that members gain from the companionship of others with similar interests during the life of the group, suggest an objective reality that requires attention.

The burden of giving care and not receiving it

Many members have defended themselves in the early meetings of the group against engaging in self-exploration, by staying in the safe role of therapist to fellow members. An even less helpful stance is as observer, in order to learn about, but not to be a member of, the group. Moving into the patient-like role of being there for oneself and for the mutual benefit of others is a significant step forward. This is not achieved by all. When it has been, it has paved the way for an examination, not without guilt and shame, of how burdensome being a carer may be and how there is a need to be directly cared for. The group experience has partially, and often helpfully, satisfied this need.

The subject matter of psychiatry is often sad and sometimes tragic. There is much struggling with the blunt implements of therapy against the unyielding clay of illness, inhibited personality and social systems. There are hard-won and surprising triumphs. For the therapist, the personal involvement and opportunity to help is both psychologically sustaining and wearing. An additional burden in caring may result from the frustration of giving to others what the therapist unconsciously wants for him- or herself, that is, the denied, needy part of self which is projected into others. The compulsive caregiver defends against this knowledge, and also against the emergence of psychotic parts of self, by denial and splitting. It is them and us, staff and patient, helper and helped – separated by a great gulf of difference. In these brief groups, it has often been possible to bridge the gulf and work with unacknow-ledged needs. What has not been reached is the 'power shadow' that Guggenbuhl (1971) depicts. In his Jungian analytic work with members of the caring professions, he has found, deeply hidden in their profes-sional shadow, a lust for power which requires the patient to submit to the therapist's domination and not achieve his or her full potential for maturity. It is likely that only in a much longer, more intimate and secure group would such dark places be reached.

Seeing others in stereotype and not as people

In the early meetings of the group, there has often been intense rivalry between the professions which replicates what has happened on wards and in multidisciplinary clinical teams. Members have had difficulty in seeing each other as people and not as stereotypes – cardboard cut-outs painted in prejudice. An uncomfortable hierarchy of doctor to psycho-logist to social worker, occupational therapist and nurse has been as-sumed by members; the assumption has historical, collusive and irrational aspects. Doctors are knowledgeable; they should lead. Nurses are ignorant academically and are condemned by themselves to be silent. Both stereotypes are unreal; both are uncomfortable and are struggled against by individuals who clearly do not fit the stereotype, but who, in the group, are caught up in its power. (Clergy should not swear but, when they do, they disrupt preconceptions and are seen as 'nice people really'.) In the membership lists for the training groups, members have been listed by name and not by title, occupation or place of work. Members have had the opportunity to divest themselves of occupational role and enter freshly into the group experience, but, interestingly, more often than not they have chosen to identify their professional role, and then regretted the misperceptions that follow. A major benefit of the group is that members come to see each other as people, and not that much different from themselves. The duration of the group allows mem-bers to check perceptions which they now recognise as misperceptions.

The training group is well placed to counter the processes of stereo-typing (Rice, 1926), self-fulfilling prophecy (Merton, 1957) and biased perception (Allport, 1937). In addition, in nearly all the groups, it has been necessary to work with the dynamic motivations that find com-fort in stereotyping. Stereotyping reduces anxiety by simplification. Fixed roles are familiar, traditional enemies are in their proper place and alliances are ready made. Negative aspects of personality can easily be split off and projected on to others, as can, conversely, idealisations.

Fear that disclosure may damage careers

Any training group run within an institution raises the fear that in disclosing personal problems or voicing criticism members of staff may damage their careers. These groups have been no exception. The fear has been noticeably evident among nursing staff, who have portrayed a hierarchical structure in their profession which is not averse to using its power punitively against its critics. The anxiety has been accentuated by superiors requiring nurse members to make a written report on the course. As Yalom has noted (1970, p. 370), when his own students attended a training group that he led, they were, to begin with, fright-ened and inhibited by him. The author has noticed similar attitudes among staff from his own institution. The issue has been partially re-solved by exploration, by making explicit the confidential nature of the group, and by using group leaders who do not work in the institution that most members come from. Now that the course is attended by personnel from all over the Trent region and beyond, the groups are more anonymous and thus less self-restricting.

When, despite all efforts to construct stranger-only groups, a group contains staff from the same ward or with some other close link, these members, and especially nurses, have tended to make an unspoken collusive pact to remain silent. They may attend in order to fulfil the commitment entered into at the beginning, but will avoid losing face by not criticising the established order, and will avoid weakening their image by not reavealing their own dilemmas. Social workers and oc-cupational therapists are less subject to this phenomenon. Neverthe-less, much disclosure does occur, events in the group and in members' lives are carefully followed, and the self-esteem of the individual, and indirectly of the group, is buoyed up by the warm interest shown by the group in these matters.

The opportunity for intimate dialogue

For some, the single most important outcome of the group is to bring them into intimate dialogue with their colleagues for the first time. One overseas doctor commented that after 2 years in England this was the first personal discussion he had had with his colleagues. When the groups work well, members reach beyond the barrier of role and give of their best. For a brief period, 10 lives unfold together. What affects one is the concern of others. For those that have engaged, the ending is a loss . . . and a chance to begin again in a new way.

Support through personal crisis and help with career decisions

Generally one or two members in each group have faced a personal crisis. Supporting their colleague through this has endowed the workings of the group with a sense of purpose. As an entity, perhaps the groups needed that gift and repaid it with care. Exploring the meaning for the member of being bereaved, ill or being admitted to hospital – the three most common crises – has meant similar exploration for other members, a reliving of old experiences, which are often given sharper edge by the symbolic significance of the group approaching its set end.

Members have used the group to take stock of where they are going in their professional and personal lives. Three areas have recurred in these reappraisals: practising psychotherapy as fully as possible, reconciling career demands when both parties in a marriage find important satisfactions in work, and adjusting to the changing roles of men and women. For members with a serious interest in psychotherapy and an inimical atmosphere at work, the choice, once the dilemmas of the institution have been more clearly understood, has been between staying and fighting for what is thought best, or leaving and embarking on a new independent venture whose parameters the therapist can define. Again, one person's decision prompts the reappraisal by others of their decisions. Male chauvinism and the assertive positions of the women's movement have been lively points of reference within the group when the relationship between men and women has come to the fore. Though members have referred to their outside relationships, the major interest has been in the actions, reactions and deductions made by one sex to the other within the group. Members have clarified their stance and been acquainted with the impression that they create. This takes up the specific requests that members frequently make in the first two meetings for feedback or help with getting in touch with feelings, being less afraid of anger and the like.

Discussion

The personal themes described in this paper arose in the context of a brief course designed to introduce inexperienced staff to the skills of leadership of therapy groups. Judging by the post-course questionnaire and the impressions of the group leaders, the training group experience is for the members the most valued component of the course. The training group is a training group and not a therapy group, though the two display more similarities than differences (Lakin, Leiberman and Whitaker, 1969; Dies, 1980); its purpose is to develop the sensitivity of members to the needs of others, to increase self-knowledge, and to deepen awareness of group processes. Whilst personal change does occur, that is not the prime purpose. It would be improper to coerce members into being patients, but the author enters one caveat to this statement: unless sufficient members enter into the patient-like role of being there for themselves, not as observers but as people with a wish to further their personal learning, the developmental potential of the group is thwarted. In the groups that have become work groups in the Bion (1961) sense of the word, at least a third of members have been active in placing their personal issues before the group, and have been supported in their actions by a further third. The silent minority has, then, remained a minority. Conversely, a silent majority sets a very different norm (Gomes-Schwartz, 1978; Fielding, 1983).

Yalom (1970) notes that in both therapy and training group members face an unknown situation in which they will be asked to expose themselves and take risks. However, training group members 'are backed up by a relatively high self-esteem level and reservoir of professional and interpersonal success. Psychiatric patients, on the other hand, may begin a therapy group with dread and suspicion. Self-disclosure is infinitely more threatening in the face of a belief in one's own worthlessness and badness' (p. 349). In the author's experience a significant minority of members have viewed their time in the group with dread and suspicion; their self-esteem has been vulnerable. Furthermore, few are without doubts about themselves and their actions. Knowing that the group will end as a unit and at a predetermined time is a considerable advantage for the training group member. In this respect, 12 weekly meetings are long enough for a worthwhile experience, but not so long as to be intimidating. Thus, some who might otherwise be frightened off are encouraged to try group work. The committed continue their training after the course by leading groups under supervision, or joining an experiential group with a longer duration.

One or two in each course of 30 do not complete the training. Sometimes these drop-outs are unwilling conscripts; sometimes they have significant personal difficulties which either are obvious once the group begins, or are activated by the experience. In addition, some have personal styles which, unless checked, are antithetical to the development of a mature group. Their management poses difficulties for the leader. The leader has no mandate to be therapist to a particular member, but equally he or she has a duty to all the members to try to ensure the richest group experience possible. The duty to the member may conflict with the duty to the group. With some, it may be possible to identify and work with the fear behind the disruptive style. One successful occasion was with a member who used his considerable powers of observation as weapons to disconcert others rather than as stepping-stones to common understanding; in so doing, he protected himself from the feared situation of assault and annihilation. On another occasion, the leader had to call a halt to the exploration of the psychopathology of a male member with a declared history of severe depression, who made repeated verbal attacks on the women in the group for attacking him, when in truth he was the provocateur. Leaders have also had to advise the group against the introduction in the closing sessions of major new issues when there was insufficient time left to explore them. As in therapy groups, members who are in the minority through some difference in race, physique, occupation or problem are at risk of isolating themselves from the group and dropping out. It should be noted that, apart from giving priority to NHS mental health staff, there is no formal selection procedure for the course. A case could be made for introducing one, but the efficiency is likely to be low. In this course, reliance has been placed upon the degree of competence of the leaders and the supervision that they give to each other after each meeting.

Leaders need a fine appreciation of what can and cannot be attempted in a brief group (Imber, Lewis and Loiselle, 1979; Poey, 1985). The 12-session limit on the duration of the group may tempt the leader to force the pace in order to achieve significant psychological work. The temptation should be resisted. A sufficient level of trust is a prerequisite for personal change and 12 weeks is a short time to build it in. Furthermore, it is both prudent for members to refrain from disclosing major areas of difficulty when the duration of the group is insufficient to sustain them in working through to new resolutions, and ethical for leaders to support them in their choice. High casualty rates have been reported among over-ambitious encounter group participants faced with charismatic, aggressive, intrusive leaders (Lieberman, Yalom and Miles, 1973). In this course, the leaders have eschewed such a style and have sought to facilitate, not manipulate (Dies, 1985); they have discouraged regressive tendencies, emphasised the capacity of members for growth, and reminded them that each is responsible for their own rate of work (Klein, 1985). The author is not aware of any casualties. Some members have been advised to seek personal therapy.

These groups have had a within-group focus. The working lives of most members are set in the context of an institution. How relevant, then, is the group experience to the professional role and is there any conflict between the two? The value of group therapy has been vividly demonstrated by the personal learning that occurs and the positive support gained from being a member of a cohesive group. The course provides direct experience of group dynamics, giving life to the theory discussed in the seminars. Group and individual processes operate in any group, whether or not it is formally constituted as a therapy group, and knowledge of these is useful whatever the work situation. However, the option of leading brief, closed small groups is often not available at work, where large group and community meetings are common practice. In recognition of this, three of the seminars in the 1986 course are devoted to a large group experience, and a further seminar to an examination of large group processes. This move capitalises on the observation that the intergroup dynamics of the training groups surface in the seminars and over supper, in the questions that members ask or do not ask of the leaders and members of the other groups. For example, rivalry may be manifested in members being willing volunteers in practicums conducted by their leader. Envy surfaces in enquiries about what goes on in the other groups, and struggles for leadership may appear in the form of displaced attacks.

Training groups for staff within a particular unit in an institution may facilitate better working relations and understanding of the patient's problems. Bennett et al. (1976) described a weekly staff group with a systems approach in a psychiatric day-hospital. There, the patient lived in two psychological and social worlds, the hospital and the external, separated to a greater or lesser extent. The staff group helped to understand the problems of the patient in the wider context by exposing the hidden family dynamics operating in the professional family system; these dynamics paralleled the patient's dymanics. While acknowledging that in this course the training groups' system is a subsystem of institutional and societal systems (Kernberg, 1975), the concern of these groups has deliberately not been with a larger system, which can only be known at one remove, and then only partially. What happens within the group can be known directly. As has been stated, when members speak of their external world, the scope for distortion through splitting is great. The temptation for the leader to collude with a 'good' group member and a 'bad' outside world is strong; conflict may be avoided and a defensive cohesiveness built. Sometimes, evidence suggests that the external criticisms are justified. Nevertheless, the group cannot judge external reality. It can, and does, deal with how a person is in the group – the reactions, the receptiveness, the matrix that is formed. This is the strength of a non-institution-linked training group. A staff group is better placed to attend to institutional issues.

The recurring themes of these groups raise issues for those concerned with the training and welfare of staff. Within the setting of a cohesive group, much useful psychological work has been possible; tragedies and sadness have been shared, the burdens of a professional role have been partially alleviated, and assistance with personal crises given. Personal learning has occurred. However, the value placed upon the experience, the anxiety expressed about seeming weak or damaging careers through disclosure, and the apparent lack of alternative settings suggest that there is a considerable unmet need for staff to be able to explore, in a setting of trust, personal issues that trouble them.

Three elements emerged from McCarley's (1975) experience with leading clinical discussion groups for 2 years, at the annual meeting of the American Group Psychotherapy Association. The first was a dominant oppressive feeling among participants of being overwhelmed by the responsibility of caring for psychiatric patients and their deep feelings of discouragement. The second was a realisation of how burdened participants have become through their dynamically urged need to give, and the third was a recognition of an inner sense of deprivation. Exploration of the last element aroused feelings of shame, which were succeeded by a reasonable acceptance that the needs of participants were as valid as those of patients. Kline (1972) has reported similar themes in a leaderless group for experienced therapists, and Berger (1967) has remarked on the active wish of therapist members to convert task-orientated groups into therapeutic experiences. Just as the injuries of life erode the confidence of patients, so may the work of psychiatry sap the morale and self-esteem of therapists. Therapists need to renew themselves; well-led groups lend themselves to this purpose.

Having leaders who are members of staff in the institutions where course members work immediately raises anxiety about the limits of confidentiality. Leaders who are independent of the work systems are at an advantage in this respect (Berger, 1967; Berman, 1975; Shapiro, 1978), However, in the author's experience, the integrity and competence of the leaders are much more important variables in facilitating the development of groups.

For some, the time in the group is one more step in their own journey of self-understanding. They know more of how their life has shaped them and developed their sensitivities. For others, their way of being in the group may demonstrate to them ways in which their personality and life experience impair their ability as therapists and which need modifying if they are to give of their best. Generally, a longer therapeutic experience is necessary for this. This consideration should be taken into account by training planners. The fact that these training groups were part of a formal skills course was important. For some, it legitimised their essay in self-exploration and avoided the stigma that might be associated with seeking personal therapy.

Again and again, members' vision of each other has been obscured by stereotyping. Once that obstacle has been surmounted, members have greatly valued the meeting in dialogue that followed. Several reports suggest that stereotyping is an important component (and hindrance) in professional working. Furnham, Pendleton and Manicom (1981), in a finding relevant to the present blurred role boundaries within multidisciplinary clinical teams, reported that each profession tends to perceive itself more positively than any other group, and perceives other professions negatively if they are in competition over a field of specialisation, a treatment method or a particular client group. Participants in a cross-hospital multidisciplinary group (Nitsun et al., 1981) gained from their contact which transcended traditional boundaries. Participants in a series of one-day workshops which examined role perceptions reached similar conclusions (Brunning and Huffington, 1985). In different language, an annual 3-day experiential–didactic workshop in psychoanalytic group therapy (Lerner, Horwitz and Burstein, 1978) promoted greater awareness of transference phenomena and empathy with the experience of patients.

The themes reported in this paper highlight the psychological world of the health care professional. The anxieties, doubts, setbacks and misperceptions will be familiar to group leaders and are recurrent. They both complicate and enrich professional work. They represent legitimate concerns, but often the institution does not attend to them. What supportive, developmental and efficiency-promoting structures should be offered? Professionals will have different requirements for depths of exploration and some problems will be specific to a setting. A reasonable provision would be threefold: first, a brief introduction to group work as a component of a training course; secondly, a 9–18 month purely experiential group, preferably with an outside leader and where members do not have close working links; and, lastly, staff groups to deal with institutional issues. Expert leadership is necessary for all three.

References

ADLER, G. (1972). Helplessness in the helpers. *British Journal of Medical Psychology* **45**, 315–325.

ALEXANDER, C. (1980) Leader confrontation and member change in encounter groups. *Journal of Humanistic Psychology* **20**, 41–55.

ALLPORT, G.W. (1937). *Personality: A Psychological Interpretation*. New York: Holt.

BENNETT, D., FOX, C., JOWELL, T. and SKYNNER, A.D. (1976). Towards a family approach in a psychiatric day hospital. *British Journal of Psychiatry* **129**, 73–81.

BERGER, I.L. (1967). Group psychotherapy training institutes: Group process, therapy, or resistance to learning. *International Journal of Group Psychotherapy* **17**, 505–512.

BERMAN, A.L. (1975). Group psychotherapy training. *Small Group Behaviour* **6**, 325–344.

BION, W.R. (1961). *Experiences in Groups and Other Papers*. London: Tavistock.

BRUNNING, H. and HUFFINGTON, C. (1985). As others see us. Altered images. *Nursing Times* 24–26 July.

DIES, R.R. (1980). Group psychotherapy: Training and supervision. In: A.K. Hess (Ed.) *Psychotherapy Supervision: Theory, Research and Practice*. New York: Wiley.

DIES, R.R. (1985). Leadership in short-term group therapy: Manipulations or facilitation? *International Journal of Group Psychotherapy* 35, 435–455.

FIELDING, J.M. (1983). Verbal participation and group therapy outcome. *British Journal of Psychiatry* 142, 524–528.

FURNHAM, A., PENDLETON, D. and MANICOM, C. (1981). The perception of different occupations within the medical profession. *Social Sciences and Medicine* 15, 289–300.

GOMES-SCHWARTZ, B. (1978). Effective ingredients in psychotherapy: Prediction of outcome from process variables. *Journal of Consulting and Clinical Psychology* 46, 1023–1035.

GUGGENBUHL, A. (1971). *Power in the Helping Professions*. New York: Spring Publications.

IMBER, S.D., LEWIS, P.M. and LOISELLE, R.H. (1979). Uses and abuses of the brief intervention group. *International Journal of Group Psychotherapy* 29, 39–49.

KERNBERG, O.F. (1975). A system approach to priority setting of intervention in groups. *International Journal of Group Psychotherapy* 25, 251–275.

KLEIN, R.H. (1985). Some principles of short-term group therapy. *International Journal of Group Psychotherapy* 35, 309–330.

KLINE, F. (1972). Dynamics of a leaderless group. *International Journal of Group Psychotherapy* 22, 234–242.

LAKIN, M., LEIBERMAN, M. and WHITAKER, D. (1969). Issues in the training of group psychotherapists. *International Journal of Group Psychotherapy* 19, 307–325.

LERNER, H.E., HORWITZ, L. and BURSTEIN, E.D. (1978). Teaching psychoanalytic group psychotherapy: A combined experiential–didactic workshop. *International Journal of Group Psychotherapy* 28, 453–466.

LEWIN, K. (1947). Frontiers in group dynamics: II. Channels of group life: Social planning and action research. *Human Relations* 1, 143–153.

LIEBERMAN, M.A., YALOM, I.D. and MILES, M.B. (1973). *Encounter Groups: First Facts*. New York: Basic Books.

McCARLEY, T. (1975). The psychotherapist's search for self-renewal. *American Journal of Psychiatry* 132, 221–224.

MALRAUX, A. (1967). Anti-memoirs. Quoted in P. Lomas (1973), *True and False Experiences*. London: Allen Lane.

MERTON, R. (1957). *Social Theory and Social Structure*. New York: Free Press.

NITSUN, M., GLEDHILL, R. and SHANLEY, R. (1981). Multi-disciplinary training groups in a psychiatric hospital. *Bulletin of the Royal College of Psychiatrists* 5, 89–91.

POEY, K. (1985). Guidelines for the practice of brief dynamic group therapy. *International Journal of Group Psychotherapy* 35, 331–354.

RICE, S.A. (1926). 'Stereotypes': A source of error in judging human character. *Journal of Personal Research* 5, 267–276.

SHAPIRO, J.E. (1978). *Methods of Group Psychotherapy and Encounter*. Itasca, IL: F.E. Peacock.

STORR, A. (1979). *The Art of Psychotherapy*. London: Secker & Warburg/Heinemann.

TUCKMAN, B.W. (1965). Developmental sequences in small groups. *Psychological Bulletin* **63**, 384–399.

YALOM, I.D. (1970). *The Theory and Practice of Group Psychotherapy*. New York: Basic Books (second edn 1975).

YALOM, I.D., BROWNS, S. and BLOCH, S. (1975). The writen summary as a group psychotherapy technique. *Archives of General Psychiatry* **32**, 605–613.

Chapter 10
Leadership in Brief Training Groups for Mental Health Care Professionals

Introduction

All applications of group psychotherapy require special expertise if they are to be beneficial in their impact. This is nowhere more true than in training groups for mental health care professionals. Such groups are a common feature of workshops, conferences and courses, and are brief in duration. The emotional significance for the participants far exceeds that which might be expected from the few hours (commonly 6–18 in total) spent together in a closed group. That the group is closed intensifies the experience, a focusing inwards which is accentuated by the detachment from external reality when the group is held in a residential setting. In this hothouse atmosphere, some group members lose their natural caution and make premature disclosures of personal history or reaction to their fellow members, which they later regret. Others may be appalled by the pace that is being set and retreat into the secure position of reticence; this is the more common pattern, especially when there is significant ambivalence to the task of the group, or simple ignorance of the personal gains that may be made through full participation. Neither response is beneficial, even though exploring the whys and wherefores of the choices that have been made is meat and drink to a group interested in the history collectively being fashioned.

The group leader has a position of responsibility. He or she is not wholly responsible for what happens during the life of the group, as this is the product of the interaction of the sovereign individuals who

From a presentation to the Xth International Congress of Group Psychotherapy, 27 August–2 September 1989, Amsterdam.

A more general version of this paper is to be found in Aveline, M.O. (1992). Principles of leadership in brief training groups for mental health professionals. *International Journal of Group Psychotherapy,* in press.

constitute its membership. Yet the role of the leader is cardinal. Much will depend on how the group is conducted, both in regard to its boundaries and its process, as these determine the group culture in which work in the Bion sense may or may not occur. Whilst the group devotee may write off to experience membership of a poorly led and unsatisfying group, the impact for the novice may be so aversive that, at worst, the mode of therapy is never again essayed or, at best, a jaundiced impression is created. Many subsequent good experiences are needed to offset a bad beginning.

This paper draws on the author's experience of leading groups in residential workshops of 3- or 5-day duration, and as a component in a 12-week introductory group course which has been held annually since 1976. After considering the leader's aims in a brief training group, and suggesting a metaphor for beneficial leadership, a number of practice points are illustrated in an account of a 12-week group.

The Aims of the Leader

The personal aims of group members can initially only be known by them. The leader has the aim of creating an environment in which the potential of the group for psychological work can be realised as fully as possible. One major constraint in brief groups is the limited time available; another is the mixed motivation of the members, a constraint that is all the more powerful as the members will not usually have been personally selected by the leader. Both constraints need to be worked with.

Being a member of a training group provides members with a learning experience about group processes, and about how they as people interact with the others that comprise this transient, but often representative, social microcosm. Although training groups are by definition not the same as therapy groups, the participants will often come to the group with the expectation of being able to raise matters of personal importance; they may reasonably hope that the experience will be therapeutic. Experienced group therapists know that being a member of a cohesive, purposeful group can be a uniquely encouraging experience in a person's life. No other therapy setting allows such opportunities for interpersonal learning through testing out how one is perceived by others, and how one's actions and inner self are received. No other setting offers such opportunities for altruistic action and the recognition and undoing of self-limiting patterns of interaction (Aveline and Dryden, 1988). In my view, the leader should aim to promote the kind of environment that will facilitate this kind of psychological work. What metaphor captures the role that I have in mind?

A Metaphor for Group Leadership

Each school of group psychotherapy has its preferred term for the therapist; each term expresses a different emphasis in practice. The orchestral
image is evoked by the group analytic *conductor*, combining and coordin-
ating the playing of individual members into a grand realisation of the
score. A less forceful image is conveyed by the *facilitator* of interpersonal group therapy. Here the therapist is more of a fellow-traveller with
group members in the journey of life; his prime task is to facilitate interaction. In gestalt therapy, the therapist is the *leader*, expressing his
central role by working with individual members one at a time, much in
the same way that Slavson and other early American therapists conducted individual analysis in a group setting. In psychodrama, the therapist is the *director*, selecting the protagonist from those who offer their
dilemmas for enactment; he sets the pace and brings the drama to a close
with de-roling and the sharing of the reverberations that have been set
off in the audience. Although a recognised style of group therapy is only
now emerging among cognitive–behaviour therapists, it is clear that for
them the very term 'therapist' contains unwelcome overtones. Instead,
the role of *educator* is preferred; skills are acquired, performance is
evaluated and homework agreed.

These terms point in different directions, but should not be taken as
being the sole description of what a group leader of a particular school
does. These are predominant emphases, with elements of the other
terms entering into the repertoire of therapy. None quite depicts the
role to which I aspire in leading brief training groups. An image from
the mountains is needed.

When walking in the high mountains with companions, I am aware
of my strength and my vulnerability. I can walk within my limits and be
safe. Yet in that safety, I may never reach hidden places or see the
sights that could be seen. In my apprehension about overextending
myself, I may needlessly underachieve. I need a guide who is familiar
with the terrain that we may traverse. The mountain guide finds out
what the party wants to do, estimates the strength of the members and
advises us when we must set out. As a member, I do not need to
concern myself with planning the route, carrying the survival equipment (except for my own whistle and waterproofs), and arranging our
transport home. I can trust in the guide and concentrate on the experience. The experience is collective, solitary and shared. No-one can
walk for me; I, myself, have to walk. From a small stumble, I pick
myself up; from a large one, others assist me. On the expedition, the
guide is even-handed in his concern, favouring neither the strongest
nor the weakest, neither setting too fast a pace nor slowing into a
debilitating dawdle. When someone falls behind, the guide drops back
to gather him or her up. The guide keeps the party together, perhaps

arranging a rendez-vous when it is safe to do so. The guide discharges his duty by being responsible and seeing the group through the difficulties *en route*. Sometimes conditions will be so dangerous that a halt will have to be called to an expedition, or a weaker member advised that a particular objective is beyond his strength.

The precise way over the mountain is set by the walkers, diverting from the path according to interest, dallying when the mood is right, and pressing on when time is short. Within limits set by time, strength and interest, the members have freedom to explore what is there to be found. In this metaphor of the group leader as a mountain guide, the terrain is not predetermined by the physical structure of an existing mountain range, but rather is formed by the members from their dilemmas, conflicts and history. It is their own nature that they explore, both in and through the collective world of the group.

Personal Themes of the Members

The short life of a brief training group imposes its discipline. For it to succeed, the group must conclude its business in the time available and its work must be cogent to the members' concerns. Yet in that time, much of personal importance may transpire. The major themes arise first from the difficulties of the professional role, and the protective barriers against vulnerability and self-doubt which are defensively imposed from within the person or projectively from without, and secondly, from the nature of human suffering and the inadequacies of the helper's response. Personal tragedies in the lives of group members, often hidden from others at work or only partially expressed for fear of being thought weak, may be expressed; the impotence of being a 'helpless helper' may be shared, and the burden of giving and not receiving may be reduced through being nurtured by the group. Members may come to recognise the stereotypes that distort their perception of each other, transcend them and the fear that disclosure may damage their careers, and meet their fellows in intimate dialogue. Other themes are to do with seeking support with personal crises and help with career decisions, especially those that conflict with parental expectations or a restrictive environment at work. The declared aim of members may be for technical instruction or academic learning, but there is usually a hidden agenda and that is personal (see Chapter 9).

Leadership Issues

Within the brief time-frame of the group the leader has five main tasks:

1. To contain the anxieties of the group.
2. To establish quickly a therapeutic atmosphere in the group.

3. To guide the group towards issues that can be addressed in the time available.
4. To guard against damaging self-disclosure and loss of self-esteem.
5. To help the group end well.

How can this be achieved? Elsewhere I have argued my preference for the interpersonal model of group therapy (see Chapter 6). The group is member-centred and has a relatively ahistorical focus on here-and-now interaction, similar to that described by Yalom (1985). This is an appropriate model for brief training groups. In addition, in the interactive space of the group I take a dialectic view of what does and does not happen. Every action is matched by reaction; whatever is done evokes the opposite, whatever is attended to means that something is not being attended to, whatever is expressed points a finger at its unspoken counterparts. The leader is well placed to attend to the unattended (as well as the usual functions of boundary-keeper, culture-former, exemplar of positive membership, historian and symbol of care-giving). The happenings of the group reflect conscious and unconscious choices made by the members. The focus on the shared experience of being in the group confirms many benefits: it is a rich source of self-understanding, clarifying as it does the characteristic ways that members interact, the important issues that through collective unconscious action might easily be avoided, and circumventing the common, invidious pressure to reveal personal secrets which often traumatises the discloser, who may then feel like a sacrificial victim, satisfying the group's need to have a patient to work with.

Examples of Leadership Issues in a Brief Training Group

In this example, disguised events from a 12-session, 12-week training group are presented. The group had ten members, seven women and three men, all health care professionals, and was led by the author. The group formed part of an introductory course in group therapy; each session was preceded by theory seminars and practicums. An unusual feature of the course is the circulation by the leader to members of a structured report on each session, and by members of their own reports after sessions 3 and 9; these reports help consolidate the work of the group and prepare members for the possible role of leader of future groups (see Chapter 14).

To ease the reader's comprehension, the course of four members, Josephine, Angela, Lawrence and Sheila, is followed in detail. Not a great deal of information is lost with this restriction, as the frequent pattern in training groups is for a third of the membership to be active in their personal and interpersonal exploration, a third intermittently so, and a third quiet. The active members, provided that together with the less active they constitute a majority of the membership, dictate the concerns and the process of the group. In this group, the fact that most of the members were women set a theme of sexuality, especially female homosexuality, which was only partially explored.

Task 1: Containing anxiety

Session 1

One member, Lawrence, was missing and no message had been received. [I opened by saying that we had 12 meetings as a group, that it was for us to decide how we used the time and that we might find it helpful to concentrate on how we related together as a group.] Josephine, a self-declared group enthusiast, quickly told the group of her fantasy that she would be eaten by sharks if she disclosed her secrets. [Her personal disclosure did not occur till session 3, but her words immediately raised the question of what she had to disclose and who she feared would be sharkish in their reply. An agenda was being set, but I stayed silent and waited to see what else would emerge.] She brought her image more in line with her direct and self-confident persona by adding that she had a shark-like self. Janice recalled being pressurised to disclose, in a previous group, her pleasure in resisting, and her ultimate sadness that she had resisted too well: an opportunity for discovery had been lost. Angela, a small delicate woman, shared her fear of being put down and indicated that her smallness of stature was an issue for her. Perhaps as a response, Sheila, a tall slim decisive woman, moved from her chair to sit on the floor, a position she occupied henceforth. This might have been comforting for Angela, but instead reminded her of men at work who took over and altered things without consultation. The move also alarmed one of the men, who was quiet and retiring in his manner. At the half-way point, a janitor put his head round the door; the group was shocked by the intrusion and reacted passively, as did I. Later, Angela surprised us by saying that she had wanted to bite his head off.

> Already a number of processes had been set going in the group. The group was interacting, a vital step towards achieving Task 2. Members were indicating what they might want to do with the time and how they did not want to be treated – not eaten, pressurised or put down – and were trying out ways of being together in the group. In a group of longer duration, it would have been possible to let the group wrestle with their fears (the reactive motive in Whitaker and Lieberman's (1964) group focal conflict model) and arrive at a solution. Brief groups, unless well managed, often get stuck with the fears and never have the chance to experience the valuable corrective of expressing their wishes and moving from a restrictive to an enabling solution. Though in itself never a

remedy for defensiveness, working on ground rules helps the group advance towards being in a position where work may be done. I set the ground rules that everyone should speak for themselves and should set their own pace, but with the expectation that the group would be a place where psychological work would be done; in this I was acting as a guide to the first steps on the terrain of the group. I promoted a discussion on confidentiality, tied to the issue of the group reports as they give visible form to what has happened in the session. The discussion helped the group to realise that it had control over its course and that, within a frame set by me as convenor, had freedom to explore the issues raised by the members.

Of the many alternative interventions, other leaders might have preferred to focus on the transference to the leader, either in the general anxiety about the leader devouring, pressurising and humiliating members, or, more specifically, about what kind of person the leader was going to be in the group. Either focus would have brought out restrictive, negative fears whose examination might have been valuable in advancing the work of the group, but which inevitably would have focused attention on the leader. In my view, having the focus on the leader is a distraction from the work that can go on between the members. Power for discovery and change primarily resides with members; the task of the leader is to help the group realise its beneficial potential. Especially in brief groups, the work is advanced by the leader showing his ethical concern through helping the group achieve a facilitative structure, rather than in highlighting the fears that inhibit the group.

Task 2: Establishing a therapeutic environment

The tasks of containing anxiety and establishing a therapeutic environment are closely related. They are worked on concurrently. Session 2 illustrates aspects of Task 2 and looks ahead to Tasks 3, 4 and 5.

Session 2

Lawrence made his debut; he depicted himself as an ambitious young professional, and was curiously concerned about having a rule of no violence in the group. [This concern left me wondering about what he feared would happen, and was the attack to come from others or from himself? My concern about his fragility and ability to work productively in the group deepened with his next remark.] He feared loss of identity in the group through not being in his work role: it meant non-existence. He showed no appreciation of the group's concern over his absence in session 1 – it was as if the first session had not occurred. In contrast, other members saw the group as an opportunity to divest themselves of occupational and social roles – to participate as a person, not as a representative of a job. Josephine, still ambivalent about disclosing her secret, introduced the image of a half-open door. The group made this image part of their evolving personal language, playing with the concept, challenging some to open their doors further and hoping that Josephine's was not locked shut. The group reports were discussed and it was agreed that they were for members' eyes only. The group was amazed to learn that at work Sheila had all her mail opened and secrets were not possible.

> I took this opportunity to bring the focus back within the group, and raised the implicit question: Were members going to force open each others' doors or read their inner secrets without permission? The group was critical of me for not being more forceful in repelling the janitor's intrusion in session 1. I accepted this criticism, both to show that I could hear the group and learn personally from what was being said about my passivity, and to be aware of the group's concern that I play my part in making the boundaries of the group as secure as possible, so that the space within could be safe.
>
> As a guide, I had to assess the strengths and vulnerabilities of members. I was already worried about Lawrence. My immediate priority was to build a therapeutic environment in the group. I encouraged members to address each other directly, speaking only for themselves and being specific; also to give and receive feedback. I used the evolving personal language of the group and took every opportunity to relate out-of-group references to within-group implied concerns, thus strengthening the identity and cohesion of the group. I avoided being drawn into one-to-one dialogues with members by drawing in others, either because they were similar in character or concern to the protagonist, or the very opposite. I made space for silent members to speak if they so wished, in order that at this stage none should be left behind in our collective journey. I endeavoured to model respect for what was said, caring for the speaker, and openness and honesty, because these are cardinal elements in a successful group.

Task 3: Guiding the group towards issues that can be addressed in the time available

Suitable issues in a brief group are:

1. The experience of each other in the group.
2. Self-assertion.
3. Owning one's own feelings.
4. Being direct.
5. Taking risks through the disclosure of feelings (not necessarily of secrets).
6. Sexuality.
7. Gaining a better sense of how one is seen by others.
8. Consensual validation and modification of perceptions.

Session 3

Josephine, after making a trial disclosure to a fellow member while being given a lift after last week, told the group that she was lesbian. 'That's that out of the way', she added. The group accepted her disclosure and made to move onto other topics.

> I openly doubted that that was that, and encouraged the group to reflect on what they and Josephine had done (the reflective loop) with the issue of her

sexuality and its implications for close feelings between women in a group where the majority were of that sex. The invitation to attend to the unattended was ignored, probably because it was too threatening for the group at this early stage in its life. Superficially, the issue was shelved and did not reappear until session 10.

Angela described her smoothing-over role in life: she was exquisitely sensitive to criticism, was under great pressure at work and had no scope to delegate any of her responsibilities. Sheila fed back that Angela seemed to view the group from behind a parapet, occasionally raising her head into view but then ducking down before she might be shot at.

> This image became part of the language of the group, a form of shorthand that all could use when Angela was in hiding, either from anticipated attack or, at a deeper level, from the emergence of her own aggressive feelings. It became an index of how well she was managing to hold her own ground in the group, to be assertive and to be sufficiently confident in her beliefs to not have to take back any opinion that she voiced. A training group cannot function well if its members merely want to observe; the personal aims of the members need to be discovered, disclosed, and the appropriate ones worked with. Angela's issue gained its urgency from its impact in her everyday life, but her recurrent self-limiting way of dealing with her conflict was played out time and time again in the group for all to see and work with.

Lawrence attracted criticism for the position he had adopted in the group. In contravention of a group decision, he had revealed his occupation, thus negating the members' wish to explore their experience of each other without the hindrance of seeing each other through the stereotypes that go with role and occupation. He complained that he was always in a no-win position, damned if he did comply, damned if he didn't. Others placed him in this position. The group became increasingly angry with him as they strove to point out that he had chosen his position; the more they pressed him, the more elusive he became. The group felt used and toyed with, as if Lawrence was playing a game to which only he knew the rules.

> I felt strongly that a familiar, negative pattern of interaction was being recreated in the group. Members were taking up their preordained roles: first Lawrence as provocateur, then members as pursuers and critics, and finally Lawrence as the lonely, misunderstood innocent whose anger was safely lodged with others through projection. However, I had no confidence that the impasse could be resolved positively for Lawrence; he could not hear what was being said and was becoming ever more fragile. I acted to guide the group away from him so as to give him a breathing space, and to present the group with a more workable focus. What roles, I asked, had members assumed when Lawrence was under pressure, and was Lawrence the only one who played games; what were they scapegoating in Lawrence that was also in themselves?

Task 4: Guarding against damaging self-disclosure or loss of self-esteem

Each session of the group presents the leader with dilemmas as to intervention, dilemmas to which there are not certain answers but where the choices that are made form the direction that the group takes. The leader has to try and fine-tune the group so that it moves neither too fast nor too slow, the former being alarming and the latter boring. Equally, the exploration in the group may be too shallow or too deep for optimal function. Emphasis may be given to concerns that turn out to be of peripheral interest, instead of central. Other dilemmas are the balance between exploring situations outside and inside the group, situations in the past and the present, and items of individual or collective interest; in all three, the latter is to be preferred. Guidance for intervention can only be tentative, as there are no absolutes in a social system whose good functioning depends on the judicious balancing of elements, each of which may or may not turn out to be beneficial, but where the result will not be known for several sessions. Each intervention needs to be tailored to the variation between groups, the strength of the members, the urgency of the need, the complexity of the problem and the duration and stage of the group. For the leader, the principal dilemmas are being too active or too passive and being too timid or too intrusive.

In sessions 4–6, Lawrence was increasingly the focus of attention. Members felt violently angry with him, the man who, intriguingly, had promoted the group rule of no violence, because of his elusive presence; he could not be pinned down over anything. He fanned the flames of rage by saying that his stance was deliberately intended, and then confused the group by accusing them of attacking him when the assault appeared to have originated with him. [I was keenly aware of the paranoid–schizoid core to his personality, and diverted the group's attention to Angela's manifest progress in being more assertive in the group.] The group appreciated her work and she appreciated being appreciated. Lawrence faded into the background, a figure to be wary of but not to be challenged.

Consequently, the group moved from a position of demoralisation to a position of self-worth, the very state that Lawrence was at heart so lacking. The demoralisation stemmed from their ineffectiveness with Lawrence, which threatened to box them into the negative solutions of either potentially shattering Lawrence by forcing their way inside him, or spiralling into ever-greater helplessness. Though my intervention may be criticised for being over-cautious, I preferred this outcome to Lawrence being damaged, or the good work that could be done with other members being obstructed by a fruitless preoccupation with him.

Perhaps unconsciously illustrating the part of Lawrence that feared intimacy, Josephine spoke of her sadness over the ending of a recent love-affair where she had been overwhelming in her affection and thus frightened away a hitherto heterosexual woman.

Again, as I noted, the theme of sexuality, especially that between women, was being raised. I chose this focus rather than the fear of intimacy because it could encompass interactions within the group, was of broad interest to members and there still remained sufficient time left in the life of the group to make a worthwhile exploration.

In session 7, Josephine recounted times when she had 'crossed the line' between friendship and sexual attraction with women, and asked the group for their reaction to what she had said. This challenged the group to examine its feelings on the subject. Beyond being reassuring about their continued positive regard for her, the group was not able to explore further. For one male member, the issue was explosive: some years before, his wife had left him for a woman; he hated her, and now doubted his masculinity. The cautionary note of this story put a brake on members' 'crossing the line' in the group. Progress was made by his being open about his ambivalence to Josephine, to whom he was attracted but who symbolised the destruction of his marriage.

Task 5: Ending well

Lawrence did not attend after session 6. First, a message was received that his father had died; later, we learnt that the father had been murdered by an acquaintaince. The group sent him a card and encouraged him to return.

Even if his father had not died and given a compelling reason for withdrawal, Lawrence's decision not to return can be seen as a self-protective act of adaptation. Although his father's death may have been a terrible demonstration of the violence that must surely have been around in his and his son's psychological world, it removed Lawrence from a situation with which he could not cope, and from which I as leader needed to protect him.

The spectres of death, loss and ending bestrode the group. Towards the end of session 7, one of the women confirmed the perception of her being sad; she had within her an unspecified lifelong sadness. This opened the way for Sheila, so confident and poised, to share her grief over the suicide of a close friend. [I reminded the group that in these endings was our ending as a group.]

The work of the group gathered pace, with much work being done on the themes of assertion, self-value and valuing, and sexuality. Angela became more able to hold her head above the 'parapet', and in session 8 deepened our understanding of the genesis of her way of coping by describing her two high-achieving, super-critical parents, whom she could neither equal in success nor please. In session 10, Sheila expressed her anger with the way in which she seemed to be being punished by her superiors for daring to leave her job after a decade of service. They either attacked her for going, or treated her as if she was already dead and gone. [How were we managing *our* ending, I asked?] Members became freer to express their appreciation of each other, balanced by a healthy anticipation of the freedom to come when the group ended. One member was encouraged not to neatly 'gift-wrap' her feelings but to give them rawly as they came. To the pleasure of all, Angela stopped being so apologetic. She could not, however, accept being given a friendly hug by Sheila; this touched on a fear of being invaded.

One of the remaining men dropped out. He had been silent throughout, despite invitations to participate actively; he responded to a message of encouragement from the group with a letter full of angry disappointment. [Neither I nor the group had understood the meaning of his silence, which in retrospect was expectant, but at the time appeared merely retiring.] In the penultimate session, two of the women and the last man shared intimate details of their histories. Their experience of sexual abuse, cruelty and prostitution made sense of their present ways of coping. In the final session, the remaining man was absent; it may be that he felt overexposed by his disclosures of the previous week. We drank some wine that Sheila brought and held to the boundary of ending at the appointed time, with no fostering of the fantasy that the group could continue in the pub. Within this frame, the issue of sexuality raised by Josephine in session 3 was returned to. For one woman, Josephine's presence had been a spur to assert her hetero-sexuality; for another, she had gained in acceptance of homosexuality, but with a knowledge that she down-played this as a potentially active constituent in her relationships; and for a third, the group had prompt-ed her to become more aware of her inner sexual confusion, an in-between state of being and, possibly, of becoming another way.

Conclusion

Brief training groups are no panacea for life's ills, but as this account demonstrates, they are not without power or value. In this example, ten strangers, all health care professionals, came together for a brief period. In their interaction they showed their characteristic patterns as particular people. They brought to the group their own concerns and, to a variable degree, worked with them. Some took a significant step forward as people. All were faced with greater awareness of them-selves. For a minority, even this gentle exploration was more than challenging enough.

Of the concerns that members bring to brief training groups, which concerns are expressed and how is a function of the group as a whole, of the issues that make up its shared history, of how liberating or frightening is their exploration in the group, and of the sequential impact of the choices that each member makes and the reverberations with past and present individual lives. A final, influential factor is the choice of route made by the leader. The leader's selective choice of route is more in the nature of a suggestion than a dictate. It draws attention to routes that could be followed and usefully explored in the time available, such as the experience of each other in the group, disclosure of feelings, self-assertion and consensual validation of perceptions (see Task 3 for a fuller list). The selective choice means that the terrain is not fully explored, some areas being left to another day. Though some members may be advised directly or indirectly against attempting a particular journey, the rest can expect that they will manage the likely hazards of the route, sustained by their confidence in the leader.

The model of leadership that I have portrayed is purposeful. It is directed towards enabling as many members of the group as possible to seize the opportunity for personal learning that the group presents. This is achieved by drawing the attention of members to the meaning of the choices that they are making (the issues addressed and ignored), and repeatedly making space for new choices in the exploration of old issues. The fact that someone interacts in the same, recurrent way with advantage or disadvantage for the quality and course of their relationships, may be brought to their attention. However, the decision to work on the pattern is theirs, and rightly so. In a brief training group, no mandate for therapy has been given, even though this may be the members' unconscious wish. The leader endeavours to create a sufficiently safe culture in the group, so that opportunities for psychological work are seen positively and taken when the time is right. This implies a gentle, almost tentative, style of leadership. Is this timidity or a proper concern for individual vulnerability in this context? In using the word 'vulnerability', is the strength of group members being underestimated and are they being deprived of what they could learn? Should the model be *not* to respect defences, but only the person within? It may be that the careful, guideship model of leadership errs on the side of caution and is at times insufficiently challenging, but I contend that it is better to have a safe, slower group than a traumatised group. Charismatic, intrusive and demanding leaders can cause havoc (Lieberman, Yalom and Miles, 1973). An encouraged but not overextended group member will want to advance his or her personal learning on another occasion.

A training group is not the same as a sensitivity group for professionals who work together. This equally demanding but little written about form of group has the purpose of improving the job performance of the members (Bramley, 1990). Training groups as I have advocated are similarly purposeful. They advance interpersonal learning and are intended to enhance the quality of relationships; they should be conducted in a constructive way. Being constructive often means being selective in what is focused on, the direction of the lead being given depending on the stage of the group, the robustness of the members and the nature of the offered foci. Lawrence's dilemmas were not those that could be addressed in a brief group; the group needed to be guided in another direction, which would help it work well and end well with no damaging loss of self-esteem for the vulnerable member. A shift into a paranoid position has lain at the core of other dilemmas requiring similar action; one example was a man who perceived himself being attacked by the women members when he was the aggressor, and who indirectly pleaded for clemency by disclosing a history of severe depression when pinpointed with his responsibility for the attacks. I remain concerned about Lawrence, and raised with him in the midgroup, written assessment of his potential for group leadership (see Chapter 14), that he consider having individual therapy. In a brief group, a key priority is to foster the healthy survival of the group as a whole, and of the individual members. To achieve this, the leader must be prepared to take effective, decisive action.

'Directive facilitation' is Dies' (1985) term for the active, supportive style of leadership that favours positive over negative interactions. In the interpersonal approach, favouring the positive over the negative is an important element. Drawing on the humanistic tradition in psychotherapy, it is nurturing that promotes growth, not criticism. The active style contrasts with the more withdrawn and detached observer-position of the group-analytic conductor, a position which if carried to the extreme can easily be experienced by the membership as punitive. Having an absent parent instead of a present guide is not what is wanted by members, who will often be unfamiliar with working in training groups and may be ambivalent about the task. The challenge of training groups is to convert observers into enthusiastic participants, the conversion of a common defensive role against interpersonal learning into an enabling solution. The here-and-now focus, the evolution of a personal language that portrays and highlights individual interpersonal issues, the prizing of the power of members to help each other, and the existential emphasis on meaning, responsibility and choice, together with a proper attention to group process and the 'unattended to' issues, all contribute to this end.

The time constraint of the brief group should not tempt the leader into the abuse of being over-directive in order to get results (Imber, Lewis and Loiselle, 1979; Poey, 1985), but equally not to intervene when disaster threatens is a dereliction of duty. The leader needs clear sight. Of course, this statement is in itself an idealisation: no-one can be so prescient or powerful that falls on the journey do not occur. My passive response to the intruding janitor (Task 1) was alarming to the group, but played a part in helping the group examine and take its own power over boundaries. Neither I nor the group were able to read correctly the expectant silence of the man who did not complete the journey of the group (Task 5). Even if we had, the result might have been the same, as he made his sovereign decision to withdraw, a right that needs to be defended in brief training groups, where for the most part the motivation of members is mixed and no screening selection has been made by the leader.

Brief training groups are no substitute for the personal learning that comes from longer membership of a group (9–18 months or more). Leadership is a skilled matter, requiring energy an a high level of professionalism – in short, the services of an expert guide. Then is the scene set for the best chance that two key features of these groups, their brevity and intensity, will be assets and not liabilities.

References

AVELINE, M. and DRYDEN, W. (1988). Group therapy in Britain: an introduction. In: M. Aveline and W. Dryden (Eds) *Group Therapy in Britain*. Milton Keynes: Open University Press.

BRAMLEY, W. (1990). Staff sensitivity groups: experiences in the field. *Group-Analysis* **23**, 301–316.

DIES, R.R. (1985). Leadership in short-term group therapy: manipulation or facilitation? *International Journal of Group Psychotherapy* **35**, 435–455.

IMBER, S.D., LEWIS, P.M. and LOISELLE, R.H. (1979). Use and abuse of the brief intervention group. *International Journal of Group Psychotherapy* **29**, 39–49.

LIEBERMAN, M.A., YALOM, I.D. and MILES, M.B. (1973). *Encounter Groups: First Facts*. New York: Basic Books.

POEY, K. (1985). Guidelines for the practice of brief, dynamic group therapy. *International Journal of Group Psychotherapy* **35**, 331–354.

WHITAKER, D.S. and LIEBERMAN, M.A. (1964). *Psychiatry through the Group Process*. New York: Atherton Press.

YALOM, I.D. (1985). *The Theory and Practice of Group Psychotherapy*, 3rd edn. New York: Basic Books.

Part III
Training and Supervision

The colour that I nail to the mast of psychotherapy training is that of effectiveness. My mongrel training and my reading of the research literature lead me to conclude that there is no one royal road to effective practice. There are a great many similar and overlapping approaches, albeit presented through widely differing languages. Part of my mission as a trainer and the originator of an NHS psychotherapy service is to try and hold together in a single service therapists of diverse orientations, in the hope that the therapies which we have now will be deployed to best effect and that a more integrated psychotherapy will emerge in the future. This will serve our patients better than the present factionalism. Of course I have a preference for one form of therapy, the interpersonal: it not only suits my personality and interest, but in my view highlights the special contribution of the psychotherapist in elucidating self-limiting patterns of relationship and working with the patient on his or her modification.

High-quality service is built on natural talent, extended by high-quality training. In both 'The training and supervision of individual therapists' and 'Issues in the training of group therapists', I take a broad, non-doctrinaire stance to training. The chapters identify key principles that may guide a novice therapist in his or her choice of training. I set out objectives in training for trainee and trainer. Since these two chapters are directed towards the great church of psychotherapy training, and not just those that are rooted in psychodynamic theory, I stress the crucial issues of countertransference and the abuse of power in psychotherapy. These issues need to be considered by all, but especially by practitioners of the more action-orientated and rational therapies, who may consider that because such dilemmas are not given prominence in their theory, they are irrelevant to their practice. This would be a blinkered view, hazardous to patient and therapist alike. Audio- and video-tape recordings are not popular with many psychodynamic psychotherapists, but they give a direct view into the consulting room, untrammelled by the vagaries of memory and the natural wish to remember events as the therapist wished they had occurred. Their use for supervision requires the highest standards of sensitivity and ethical behaviour from the therapist ('The use of audio- and video-tape recordings in the supervision and practice of dynamic psychotherapy').

Much of my effort over the years has been directed towards finding new ways that will enhance the opportunity for learning that psycho- therapy presents. For several years, I used to mail a written report to members of my therapy groups after each session, as a way of replaying the meeting and underlining its value. A similar technique is described in 'The use of written reports in a brief group psychotherapy training', wherein trainee group therapists have their powers of observation strengthened by writing and receiving structured reports on sessions in which they have been participant members. 'The Nottingham experi- ential day in psychotherapy: a new approach to teaching psycho- therapy to medical students' describes a personal, active approach to learning, in which the students learnt about psychotherapy through learning about themselves.

No service or training scheme can function well without a critical mass of experienced therapists who subscribe to a common purpose. 'Developing a new NHS psychotherapy service and training scheme in the Provinces' charts what can be done within the NHS over 17 years in an area with no established tradition of psychotherapy provision. I hope that it may serve as a blueprint for others in the same position to consider when dreaming their dream and planning their service.

Chapter 11
The Training and Supervision of Individual Therapists

The purpose of training in psychotherapy is to facilitate the exercise of natural abilities and acquired skills to best effect. This statement, which is based on my experience as a trainer in psychotherapy in the National Health Service, asserts two propositions, each of which is central to this chapter. First, that therapists bring to their work a greater or lesser degree of natural talent for psychotherapy. Two subsidiary propositions are that the possession of talent is an essential foundation on which expertise can be built in training, and that the talent is not a unitary predisposition; the talent may be for one of the individual therapies or for some other form such as group or family therapy. Second, that psychotherapy is a purposeful activity in which trainees and trainers share a professional and ethical commitment to evaluate and refine their work. Thoughtful therapists will ask themselves three questions again and again: What in the therapy and this person's life actually helped the patient? Could the end have been achieved more expeditiously? Was anything done that was to the patient's ultimate detriment? (In this chapter 'the patient' is a generic term for someone who suffers and is seeking help.)

In this chapter it is impossible to do justice to the fine detail of training in each of the many forms of individual therapy. Instead, attention is drawn to important issues in each area of training. After the introduction, I present a checklist of training objectives, then proceed to discuss motivating factors in therapists and selection for training, before considering the sometimes neglected but universally important dimensions of countertransference and the abuse of power. The three cardinal elements of theoretical learning, supervised clinical work and

From M.O. Aveline (1990). The training and supervision of individual therapists. In: W. Dryden (Ed.) *A Handbook of Individual Therapy*, pp. 313–339. Milton Keynes: Open University Press.

personal therapy are discussed in turn. Supportive therapy and the need for continued education are then considered. A section on the registration of psychotherapists completes the overview.

Introduction

'In what is called "individual psychotherapy", two people meet and talk to each other with the intention and hope that one will learn to live more fruitfully.' This deceptively simple statement by Lomas (1981, p. 5) encompasses the central dimensions in psychotherapy practice – meeting, talking (I prefer the form 'talking with' rather than 'talking to') in a hopeful spirit and the purposeful intention of achieving more fruitful living in the patient's everyday life. The statement sets out in ordinary language the parameters of a kind of psychotherapy with which I can identify, a rather ordinary encounter between two people, but one of exceptional promise. However, as is so often the case, the results of our intentions frequently do not measure up to our hopes. Training is intended to enhance the competence of the therapist but in itself is no guarantee of success. Please note that trainings which emphasise the apparent substantial difference in form between therapies may obscure underlying, powerful similarities.

Luborsky, Singer and Luborsky (1975), in a survey of the effectiveness of different approaches to psychotherapy subtitled 'Is it true that "everyone has won and all must have prizes"?', calls attention to the fact that all the psychotherapies are similarly effective and none preeminent, a sobering conclusion for partisans of their school or faction. In other words, what effective therapies across schools have in common is more important than what divides them – a theme I return to later. This is not to say that certain therapies are not particularly suitable for a given person or problem, nor that a therapist will not function especially well in the approach that he or she finds most congenial. What are the best applications of the different therapies is a matter for research, while the natural affinity of a trainee for particular approaches is a key aspect to be identified in training.

The findings of Luborsky and other researchers certainly have not stilled debate about who is or is not a psychotherapist, or which theoretical system if any contains the most truth. Or can one variant, for example psychoanalysis and psychoanalytic psychotherapy which share so many features, consistently and with enhanced therapeutic effect, be distinguished from the other? Sandler (1988), a distinguished psychoanalyst, thinks not. In such debates, questions of power, prestige and authenticity lurk in the shadows and threaten to upstage the essential questions of how appropriate and effective are the approaches with which patients and what problems. All the warring tribes in the psychotherapy nation have a vested interest in promoting their ascendancy over competitors and, within their own ranks, in stilling dissident voices; in such struggles, the pursuit of truth may be neglected. In selecting a training programme, trainees need to bear these points in mind.

Given the wide range of approaches that may be gathered under the generic title of individual psychotherapy, and the partisanship that goes with differences that are often more apparent than real, I am mindful of the hazard of this chapter being dismissed by adherents of one approach on the grounds of irrelevance to their practice, ignorance of what they do or believe, and partiality to my own bias. In contrast, my intention is to address important issues for trainees *and* trainers, which I hope will be heard across the spectrum. But first I must state what is central to my approach for two reasons. I will be declaring my bias and setting out a synthesis, derived from my experience as a therapist, with which the reader may compare his or her own conclusions.

Psychotherapy attends both to the vital feelings of hope, despair, envy, hate, self-doubt, love and loss that exist between humans, and to the repeated pattern of relationships that a person forms; in particular, to those aspects of the patterns for which that person has responsibility and over which they can come to exercise choice. As a therapist, I encourage my patients to take personally significant action in the form of new ways of relating, both in the consulting room and in their relationships outside, that, once succeeded in, will begin to rewrite the cramped fiction of their lives. This therapeutic action challenges the determining myths that individuals have learnt or evolved to explain their actions; commonly, these myths are restrictive and self-limiting. I work with the psychological view that people take of themselves, their situation and the possibilities open to them; essentially, this is the view that has been taken of them by important others, and by them of themselves in the past, and which will go on being the determining view unless some corrective emotional experience occurs (Aveline, 1986). The view that individuals take of themselves is illuminated by the relationship patterns that form between patients and the people in their lives and me; jointly, the patient and I examine the meaning of the patterns. Importantly, it is change in the external world of the patient, rather than inferred intrapsychic change, against which I judge the success of our mutual endeavour. Lest this sound too demanding, let me balance the statement by the recognition that many with deep problems of self-doubt and negative world view need sustained care in order to gather the courage to change.

On one level, I make no distinction between enlightened analytic and behaviour therapy that both recognises and utilises the therapeutic factors they have in common; they both offer encouragement, the one covertly, the other overtly. In the former, intrapsychic terrors are faced and the treatment proceeds by analogy; if a new end to the old sad story can be written in the relationship with the therapist, the same new chapter can be written in the natural relationships outside the consulting room. In the latter, direct action is taken, perhaps after a period of rehearsal, often undertaken with the therapist. What characterises good psychotherapy of any sort is a sustained, affirmative stance on the part of an imaginative, seasoned therapist who respects and does not exploit (Schafer, 1983). I hope that my relationship with the patient is both passionate and ethical, for both these elements are necessary if personal change is to occur. In the interplay of therapy, I influence and am influenced by what passes between us. It is the other person's journey in life, but it is a journey for us both and one in which I may expect to change as well as the patient. It is a journey and not an aimless ramble; though the ultimate destination may be unknown, the way-stations are known and aimed for; the therapist has expertise in guiding the other through terrain which is novel for them. It is also a journey in which I do not expect to be the guide for the whole way; someone may enter therapy for a while, gain what they require to get their life moving, go away to try their modified approach and return later if they need; in this, I am a minimalist. I do not aim, even if it were possible, as early psychoanalysts hoped, to exhaust through the therapy the patient's potential for neurosis or, necessarily, to place the locus of change wholly in the relationship with me.

I have presented my conclusions in summary form. The constraint of space means that I cannot spell out the significance of each point, but I offer my conclusions as a personal point of reference for the following discussion of the elements in training. Let us begin by recognising the formidable task that awaits the trainee therapist.

What the Individual Therapist Has to Learn

Despite the plethora of texts and manualised procedures whose purpose is to lend assistance to both experienced and novice therapists, the practice of psychotherapy is challenging in its elusive complexity, ambiguity and frustratingly slow pace of change. Even in the more procedure-dominated cognitive and behavioural therapies, the ambiguous, uncertain reality of practice is disconcerting to those (and this includes many with medical, nursing and psychology backgrounds) who are used to the predictable clarity in the physical sciences of structure, intervention and consistent outcome. Furthermore, what happens between therapist and patient is complicated by the often unrecognised involvement of the therapist in the patient's self-limiting fiction, and by the arousal in the therapist of unresolved personal conflicts; this phenomenon of transference and countertransference has the central place in the analytic therapies (and, of course, is fostered by their techniques) but, to a greater or lesser extent, is also part of any human interaction, and certainly of any therapy where the participants have a close relationship. Yet, I trust, for readers of this volume the struggle to become proficient as therapists is worthwhile, not least because psychotherapy is a fundamentally important activity in our technological and materialistic age; it attends to individual and shared experience and meaning and it attests to the ability of people to support and help each other. But this practical discipline and creative art is not easily learnt.

What a therapist has to learn depends on the level and intensity at which he or she has to practise, be it at the level of beginners gaining a limited appreciation of what psychotherapy is, or of qualified professionals who as generalists need psychotherapeutic skills as part of their work, or of career psychotherapists and future trainers of therapists. The caveat to this is that, at all levels, the same lessons are repeated again and again. The individual therapies vary substantially in theory, focus and technique and there is much to be learnt. However, the trainee who quite appropriately immerses him- or herself in one approach risks being ignorant of other approaches. It is thus tempting when faced with such variety to attempt to learn simultaneously two dissonant approaches, but trainee confusion and trainer alienation may result. Yet not to look widely at the therapy spectrum during the formative period of training is to risk premature closing in thinking, and mental ossification.

General objectives for the trainee therapist

1. To make progress towards the optimal use of natural ability and acquired skills.
2. To identify the type(s) of therapy and range of patient problem and personality with which the therapist can work effectively.

Specific objectives (in approximate order of priority)

1. To learn to listen to what is said and not said by patients, and to develop with them shared languages of personal meaning.
2. To develop the capacity to keep in contact with patients in their pain- and anger-filled explorations.
3. In interaction with patients, to learn to move between participation and observation. To get a sense of when and when not to intervene.
4. To gain a coherent conceptual frame with which to understand what happens and is intended to happen in therapy.

5. To study human development, the process of learning, and the functioning of naturally occurring personal relationships between friends, couples and in families, and the artificial, constructed relationships in psychotherapy where strangers are brought together.

6. To understand and bring to bear both the therapeutic factors that types of therapy have in common (these, which are often referred to as non-specific factors, are detailed in the section on theoretical learning) and those that are approach-specific.

7. To gain confidence in the practice of the preferred type of therapy. To make full use of one's own emotional responses, theoretical constructs and techniques in resolving the patient's problems.

8. To increase one's own level of self-awareness and to work towards the resolution of personal conflicts which may interfere with the process of therapy.

9. To come to know personal limitations and be able to obtain and use supervision.

10. To know the features of major psychiatric illness and the indications and contraindications for psychotropic medication.

11. To make valid diagnostic assessments psychiatrically, psychologically and dynamically (Malan, 1979, Chapters 17–22).

12. To be sufficiently knowledgeable about other types of therapy so as to match optimally, by referring on, patient and approach (and therapist).

13. To consider ethical dilemmas and internalise high ethical standards.

14. To cultivate humility, compassion and modesty as well as a proper degree of self-confidence.

15. To be familiar with the chosen theoretical system and aware of its areas of greatest utility and its limitations. To appreciate the significance of cultural and social factors, and to adjust therapy accordingly.

16. To evaluate critically what is enduring truth and what is mere habit or unsubstantiated dogma in the practice of psychotherapy, through the experience of clinical practice, being supervised and studying the research literature.

17. At the level of career psychotherapist, to acquire that professional identity.

Objectives for the trainer

1. To assess accurately both the stage at which trainees are in their development as therapists, and their strengths and weaknesses. At different stages, this may involve the normative functions of selec-

tion for training and evaluation for graduation. (In educational terms, 'normative' refers to entry/exit, pass/fail criteria, whereas 'formative' refers to non-examined elements that enrich the educational experience of training.)

2. To help trainees secure the formative learning experiences which will clarify and develop their natural affinity for particular types of therapy and problem.

3. To hold the balance of interest between the learning needs of trainee therapists and the clinical needs of their patients, until such time as the trainee therapists can do this for themselves.

This long list is not intended to be intimidating but it does serve to underline the seriousness of embarking on training to be a therapist. It provides a framework with which to assess training needs, progress, and the suitability of the training programme for a particular trainee.

Training has no end-point or single path. An individual's training over time is the result of personal and occupational choices. The choices may mark a progression from the expertise needed by a generalist with an interest in the subject, to that required by a career psychotherapist, and within psychotherapy from one type to another as the trainee's interest changes. Just as therapy should meet the needs of the patient, so should training meet the requirements of the therapist's practice, stemming both from the type of therapy and from the work setting. Thus, what a therapist working in brief therapy in a clinic with a long waiting list needs to know is very different from one specialising in long-term therapy in independent practice, who takes on new work only when he or she has a vacancy.

The reader at this point may be eager to plunge into the detail of the three cardinal elements of training, namely theoretical learning, supervised clinical work and personal therapy. To accede to this wish would be premature. It would collude with the view that proficiency in psychotherapy is a simple acquired skill. Instead, I argue that the wish to train in psychotherapy arises from events in the trainee's personal history and their consequent effect on character structure. The reflective therapist will want to take stock of what he or she brings from his or her inheritance and experience of life to this work, before he or she becomes deeply committed to it. Two things are certain. In the work of psychotherapy, whatever the type, the personal, unique reactions of the therapist will complicate and illuminate the relationship with the patient, and will expose him or her to the temptation of abusing the powerful position of therapist. What I mean by these strong statements is spelt out in the next four sections, which deal with motivating factors in the therapist, the selection of therapists for training, countertransference and the abuse of power.

Motivating Factors in the Therapist

The trainee therapist has been long in the making before he or she formally enters training. Family circumstance, life events, gender, race and culture combine with inherited predisposition to form a unique individual, who may or may not be suited to the practice of some or all ofthe psychotherapies. Individual potential therapists will be special in their values, expectations and sensitivities; each will have natural ability in different measure for the work, and natural affinity for particular types of therapies and patient problems.

Being a psychotherapist has many satisfactions: the opportunity to develop a unique personal style of practice with a substantial degree of professional independence, to share at close hand an endless variety of human activities far beyond that generally encountered in the therapist's own life, to satisfy the desire to help others, to be intellectually stimulated, to gain in emotional growth, . . . and to have prestige and be paid! (Burgental, 1964; Burton, 1975; Greben, 1975; Farber and Heifetz, 1981; Farber, 1983).

Guy (1987) distinguishes between functional and dysfunctional motivators. In fact, his items encompass both motivating factors and functional attributes of effective therapists. Functional motivators include a natural interest in people, the ability to listen and talk, the psychological-mindedness of being disposed to enter empathically into the world of meaning and motivation of others, and the capacities of facilitating and tolerating the expression of feelings, being emotionally insightful, introspective and capable of self-denial, as well as being tolerant of ambiguity and intimacy and capable of warmth, caring and laughter (see also Greben's (1984) six functional attributes on pp. 166–167).

Dysfunctional motivators draw people to the role of therapist and *may* prove to be functional, but when present to excess subvert the process for the therapist's own ends. There is a well-established tradition in dynamic psychotherapy, clearly articulated by Jung, that only the wounded healer can heal. Thus, Storr (1979) writes 'Psychotherapists often have some personal knowledge of what it is like to feel insulted and injured, a kind of knowledge which they might rather be without but which actually extends the range of their compassion'. Guy (1987) lists six dysfunctional motivators of which the first is the most common:

1. Emotional distress, where therapists may seek – and gain – self-healing through their work; the crucial question is one of magnitude. Some acquaintance with emotional pain is essential; an over-preoccupation with unresolved personal needs hinders the therapist from giving full attention to the patient.
2. Vicarious coping as a lifestyle which imparts a voyeuristic quality to the therapy relationship.

3. Conducting psychotherapy as a means of compensating for an inner sense of loneliness and isolation: this is self-defeating as it is life lived at one remove.
4. Fulfilling the desire for power and fostering a false sense of omnipotence and omniscience (Marmor, 1953; Guggenbuhl-Craig, 1979).
5. A messianic need to provide succour; one positive aspect of psychotherapy is that it is an acceptable way for people to show their love and tenderness, but this becomes dysfunctional when it is carried to excess.
6. Psychotherapy as a relatively safe way of expressing underlying rebellious feelings in the therapist through getting the patient to act them out.

These dysfunctional motivators give rise to countertransference problems, which are considered later. (Countertransference means distortions derived from unresolved conflicts in the therapist's life which he or she unconsciously introduces into the therapy relationship.)

The prevalence of dysfunctional motivators among psychotherapists is not known. In a major survey of 4000 American psychotherapists (Henry, 1977), most reported good relationships with their families, though in 39 per cent their parents' marriage was not good. Childhood separations, deaths and incidence of mental illness were similar to that of other college-educated populations. These global statistics doubtless conceal much individual variation. Thus Storr's (1979) impression may be true that many therapists (and here he means dynamically oriented therapists) have had depressed mothers to whose feelings they may have developed a special sensitivity, together with an urge not to upset or distress; their childhood experiences may well have prompted them to seek out in adult life the role of therapist. In Kleinian terminology, the need to make reparation will be great in these therapists; they may be especially adept in making contact with timid and fearful patients. There is some evidence that within the occupation of psychotherapy a history of personal conflicts and a greater experience of mental illness in their family of origin inclines practitioners more towards dynamic rather than behavioural orientations (Rosin and Knudson, 1986). I know of no research that distinguishes between the personal backgrounds of therapists choosing to work in individual therapy and those choosing family and group therapy.

These factors and attributes constitute the natural ability for which selection has to be made and which is built on in training.

The Selection of Therapists for Training

Trainers have a dual responsibility in selecting their trainees. The responsibility to the trainee is to help that person to avoid taking on work for which he or she is not suitable *and* to the patients from whom he or she will learn, to ensure that they have optimal care.

Selection is a matter for both the trainee and the trainer; the trainee will want to test out what is on offer and the trainer will test the trainee's readiness for each level of training. Introductory trainings, through workshops and brief courses, offer the trainee the opportunity to try different types of therapies and to discover the ones for which he or she has a natural affinity. Little or no attempt is made to select at this level. Another formative route into formal psychotherapy training is to be supervised by therapists whose style and orientation vary and, either before or as a supplement to this, to be in personal therapy; both experiences form and clarify aptitude. With advancing level, selection procedures become correspondingly complex. Commonly, for analytic training, candidates will have to complete an autobiographical questionnaire and undergo two extended interviews with different assessors, one more factual and the other explorative in the analytic style; the results will be considered by a panel of assessors, so as to reduce individual bias (a detailed explication of the process and criteria used in one institute can be found in Fleming, 1987, Chapters 3 and 7). Later, the candidate's progress will have to be approved before entry to each further stage of training is allowed.

Sadly, the correlation between training and effectiveness as a therapist is low (Auerbach and Johnson, 1977); this finding may reflect deficiencies in research methodology, but is also a function of the overwhelming importance in promoting personal change of pre-existing personality factors such as decency, a respectful empathic concern with others, neutrality, persistence and optimism. To continue this diversion into research, effectiveness as a therapist over the years often follows a U-curve and is a function of different attributes; early on, patients benefit especially from the therapist's energy and enthusiasm, and later from acquired wisdom and skill as a therapist. In the middle phase, as therapists become more self-conscious and aware of the complexity of the subject, performance may decline temporarily. Trainees should not feel dismayed by feeling deskilled when they enter the next level of training, and may with justice on their side ask the training organisers what help they propose to provide with this common reaction.

The above should not be taken to imply that putting effort into selection is worthless. Personality is all-important. 'The greatest technical skill can offer no substitute for nor will obviate the pre-eminent need for integrity, honesty, and dedication on the part of the therapist' (Strupp, 1960). As a selector, I look for the functional motivators listed by Guy (1987) but, also, the six qualities identified by Greben (1984): empathic   concern,   respectfulness,   realistic   hopefulness,   self-awareness, reliability and strength – for these are the qualities that are necessary if the therapist is to win the patient's trust; they give him or her the sense of being tended to and valued. Women often seem to have these qualities in greater abundance then men. It must be stressed that no-one is perfect; what is required for this work is a sufficiency of these qualities. In addition, I look for two markers of maturity in life; first, that the trainee has struggled with some personal emotional conflict and achieved a degree of resolution, and second, has enjoyed and sustained over years a loving, intimate relationship. The first may bring in its wake humility and compassion, the second an active commitment to and capacity for good relationships, so well summed-up in Fairbairn's (1954) concept of mature dependence. I am wary of aspiring therapists who have a scornful, rejecting or persecutory cast to their nature, or who are not emotionally generous in their interaction.

My impression is that therapists who prefer to work in individual therapy rather than in, for example, group therapy have a number of identifying characteristics. They seem to have a greater interest in the vertical or historical axis of there-and-then exploration into the childhood origins of adult problems and their recreation within the therapy relationship, as opposed to the horizontal axis of here-and-now interactions which is central to the focus of the group therapist (and increasingly of the modern psychodynamic therapist). They are more interested in fantasy, prefer to take a passive role and like the immediacy of the one-to-one relationship and the scope to work in depth. These impressions may help the trainee in the choice of which type of therapy to train in, though other factors will also be influential. The high patient demand for individual therapy and its greater economic viability in private practice may powerfully reinforce a natural affinity for the dyadic way of working.

A controversial issue concerns whether or not a trainee therapist should have, as a prerequisite for being a psychotherapist, a qualification in one of the core health care professions; these are generally taken to be medicine, psychology and social work, all degree occupations, but should also include nursing and occupational therapy and, perhaps, the new categories of art and drama therapy. Talent as a psychotherapist is not the exclusive preserve of any profession. However, the possession of a core qualification indicates that the trainee has a certain level of intelligence and ensures familiarity with the symptoms and signs of major psychiatric illness. It will also have offered the trainee the opportunity to internalise high ethical standards and, through membership of a professional organisation, ensures that he or she will be subject to disciplinary procedures which help maintain good practice. Qualifications in literature, philosophy and religion are relevant, but trainees with these backgrounds will need special training in the features of major psychiatric illness and what may be gained from pharmacological treatment, especially if they intend to practise independently. I shall return to this question in the sections on theoretical learning, supervised practice and registration.

In the foregoing two sections I have written at some length about the personal qualities and qualifications that a trainee therapist brings to the work. In order to bring out two important consequences that stem from the intensity of the closed, asymmetrical personal relationship between patient and therapist that lies at the heart of individual therapy, the next two sections deal with the importance of countertransference reactions and the temptations for therapists to abuse their power in *all* types of psychotherapy.

Countertransference

Unconsciously mediated transference and countertransference reactions inevitably feature in any relationship, and especially in the intimate, prolonged relationship of individual therapy. Even in the symptom-oriented, individual cognitive and behaviour therapies, these powerful distortions are present. However, many behavioural training programmes pay scant attention to these processes, a deficiency shared by some more psychodynamically based individual therapies. Trainees are advised to check that attention is given in the training to this aspect of the therapy relationship.

Individual therapists need to be as fully aware as possible of how these distorting processes are operating, what they may mean and what implications they may have for the work. Let us illustrate this with the consequence of a positive transference reaction in two types of individual therapy; in this reaction, the patient may transfer on to the therapist idealised, dependent feelings which derive from the relationship with his parents, but which may also signify an unresolved intrapsychic conflict and a dependent style in relationships. In a supportive psychotherapy in which, by definition, deep probing of mental defences and conflicts is avoided, the consequence of understanding what was happening might be not to address and try to resolve the transference but simply to bear in mind the hazard of fostering unnecessary dependence and to make use of the transference in mobilising the patient's sense of hope and expectation of benefit from the therapy. In behaviour therapy, the passive compliance that signifies that a person may not have mastered the maturational task of separation and individuation would be understood for what it means, probably not addressed on the level of its historical significance, but circumvented by encouraging the patient to take the initiative in devising behavioural tasks. Of course in the analytic therapies, directly examining these reactions and counterreactions is the focus of the work.

The term 'countertransference' is used in two senses: it may refer both to feelings that are the counterpart of the patient's feelings and to feelings that are counteractions to the patient's transference (Greenson, 1967). Counterpart feelings are part of empathy; they provide valuable information about the other, as when the therapists feels in him- or herself the disowned, hidden sadness or anger of the other. Thus the therapist's unconscious mind understands that of the patient (Heimann, 1950). Counteractions are situations where the patient's communications stir up the unresolved problems of the therapist. An example would be a therapist who fears his or her own aggression and placates the patient whenever hostile feelings are detected. In addition, the patient, through some combination of age, gender or other characteristics, may be a transference figure for the therapist; examples would be as parent or rival. Furthermore, the dependence and intimacy of the role relationship of therapist and patient will have a personal meaning for the therapist, based on past and childhood experiences of psychologically similar situations.

Consider the following list of countertransference reactions and their consequences (Bernstein and Bernstein, 1980), and see how each limits the therapeutic potential of the encounter.

1. Do I require sympathy, protection and warmth so much myself that I err by being too sympathetic, too protective toward the patient?
2. Do I fear closeness so much that I err by being indifferent, rejecting, cold?
3. Do I need to feel important, and therefore keep patients dependent on me, precluding their independence and assuming responsibility for their own welfare?
4. Do I cover feelings of inferiority with a front of superiority, thereby rejecting patients' need for acceptance?
5. Is my need to be liked so great that I become angry when a patient is rude, unappreciative or uncooperative?
6. Do I react to patients as individual human beings or do I label them with the stereotype of a group? Are my prejudices justified?
7. Am I competing with other authority figures in the patient's life when I offer advice contrary to that of another health professional?
8. Does the patient remind me too much of my own problems when I find myself being overly ready with pseudo-optimism and facile reassurance?
9. Do I give uncalled-for advice as a means of appearing all-wise?
10. Do I talk more than listen to patients, in an effort to impress them with my knowledge?

Countertransference problems are signalled by intensifications or departures from the therapist's usual practice. At the time, they seem plausible, even justifiable, yet when considered in supervision or in the routine self-scrutiny that is the mark of responsible psychotherapy, their obstructive nature becomes apparent. Menninger (1958) lists among the items that he has 'probably experienced': repeatedly experiencing erotic feelings towards the patient, carelessness in regard to appointment arrangements, sadistic unnecessary sharpness in formulating interpretations, getting conscious satisfaction from the patient's praise or affection, and sudden increase or decrease in interest in a certain case.

Items like the above serve as a checklist to help identify countertransference problems that arise from conflicts in the therapist's unconscious mind. This is different from the equally problematic feelings that are manifestations of the therapist's involvement in the patient's determining fiction or, in the language of psychoanalysis, the transference and transference neurosis; one example would be the way in which a patient who has been brought up in a persecutory environment expects others to persecute him or her, perceives the therapist as being persecutory (transference) and prompts the therapist actually to act in a persecutory way (transference neurosis); another example would be when the therapist finds him- or herself not respecting the boundaries of a patient whose childhood boundaries were breached by a parent in incestuous acts. A golden route for promoting change lies in identifying these involvements, exploring their meaning and disentangling both therapist and patient from them. Both sets of involvements are encompassed within a new taxonomy of therapist difficulty devised by Davis et al. (1987). This allows therapists to compile their own distinctive profile of difficulty on nine categories. Trainees might benefit from plotting their profile and using this to highlight to them their idiosyncracies, which could then be focused on in training.

The Abuse of Power

A particularly common form of noxious therapy relationship results from the abuse of power. Individual therapists are all too easily seduced into abusing the therapy relationship. When this occurs, the relationship is no longer therapeutic. During training, trainees need to learn how to recognise when abuse is likely to happen and is happening, and take corrective action. In this respect, the work that is done in supervision is crucial. How does the abuse of power come about? It results from the conjunction of the patient's transference wishes and dysfunctional motivators in the therapist; it is encouraged by the inequality of power between the two.

The arena in which individual therapy takes place is constructed essentially by the therapist. Though subject to negotiation, the therapist decides the duration frequency and form of the therapy. Ultimately, beginning and ending is in his or her hands, the latter being a powerful threat to the patient who is dependent or not coping. With rare exception, the meeting takes place on the therapist's territory. The therapist, whether trainee or trained, is held to be expert in what goes on in the arena, certainly by the patient, who is relatively a novice in this setting. What procedures the therapist propounds, the patient is predisposed to accept. Because the sessions take place in private, the therapy is not subject to the natural regulation of the scepticism and even incredulity of outsiders. All this gives therapists great power, and consequently exposes them to great temptation.

Ideological conversion through a process analogous to brainwashing is one hazard. When Scientology was investigated (Foster, 1971), its practices of 'auditing' and 'processing' were seen to be so dangerous that statutory regulation of psychotherapy was called for. More commonly, eccentric unsubstantiated beliefs are peddled as truths, and clung on to by vulnerable, uncertain people who deserve better.

Another hazard for the patient is the conjunction of the patient's need for an ideal parent who will protect, guide and succour with the therapist's wish to be idealised. What Ernest Jones (1913) termed the 'God complex' lies in wait for the unwary (Marmor, 1953). The therapist's ego is boosted by transference admiration; this seductive pitfall is compounded by the common tendency in psychotherapy, and especially in individual therapy, for therapists to mystify the process through the use of esoteric jargon and the adoption of an aloof, all-knowing stance. Therapists run the risk of coming to feel superior, free from the struggles, conflicts and defeats of their patients. From a detached position, which may be bolstered by viewing all the patient's communications as manifestations of transference and, as such, needing only to be put back to the patient for his sole consideration, the therapist is tempted to be a bystander on life, vicariously involved but spared the pain and puffed up by the patient's dependent approval. Progress towards separation and individuation is obstructed. In the artificial, time-limited world of the therapy session, the therapist may have the pretence of having all the answers.

Guggenbuhl-Craig (1979) asserts that within us all is the archetype of the patient and healer. In order to reduce ambivalence, the archetype may be split and either polarity projected on to others, but both are necessary for healing. The sick man needs an external healer, but also needs to find the healer in himself; otherwise he becomes passive through handing over his healing ability to the other. This is obviously antithetical to the spirit of good psychotherapy. For the healer, the danger is to locate the polarity of the 'patient in himself' in the patient and not recognise it in him- or herself. He or she will then come to see him- or herself more and more as the strong healer for whom weakness, illness and wounds do not exist. As a healer without wounds, he or she will be unable to engage the healing factor in the patient. Traditional medical education can reinforce this division (Bennett, 1987).

The therapist who locates weakness in others becomes powerful through their failure. In Jungian language, the charlatan shadow of the therapist has been constellated. Guggenguhl-Craig (1979) doubts that personal therapy or case discussion is sufficient to reduce the split in the archtetype. The analytic shield carefully acquired in training is too effective, the risk of loss of self-esteem or prestige too great, the need to maintain one's allegiance to a school of therapy against outside attack too pressing. In some therapists, the split in the archetype is minimal; their patients' problems illuminate their own, and are consciously worked on; they remain a patient as well as a healer. The best way of reducing the split is through involvement in ordinary life in unanalytical, symmetrical relationships which have the power to touch deeply, and to throw off-balance, relationships which are quite different from the asymmmetrical ones of therapy. Friendships – loving, forceful encounters with equals – develop the therapist as a whole person. What the therapist advocates for others is good for him- or herself.

Not surprisingly, given the intensity and privacy of individual therapy, some therapists become sexually involved with their patients. It is hard to conceive of circumstances when this is not abusive in its impact, or when it is not a dereliction of the responsibilities of being a therapist. One can understand how it happens but it should not be condoned. Many more male therapists have sexual involvements with female patients than do female therapists with male patients, but all combinations do occur, including with the same sex. Eroticised transferences and countertransferences are common in therapy and may be acted out (Holroyd and Brodsky, 1977). In the transference, the patient may be looking for a loving parent. This wish may connect with the therapist's need to be a helping figure, but subsequent sexual action represents a confusing of childhood wishes, albeit expressed in adult language, with mature intent; sexual action disregards the boundaries that are necessary if the therapy arena is to be psychologically safe.

Lust is a relatively straightforward motivation in acting out; its intensity depends on the urgency of the therapist's biological drive, age, state of health, recency of drive satisfaction, general satisfaction with personal life and, of course, the attractiveness of the patient. Darker motivations such as unconscious hostility towards women, or reaction-formations against feared homosexuality or gender inadequacy, may be present (Marmor, 1972). Sexual action may be rationalised as being for the patient's benefit, but this self-deception should not survive the monitoring of self-scrutiny, supervision and personal therapy.

Occasionally, therapist and patient fall in love and form a long-term relationship. Though one may wonder about the basis of a personal relationship founded in the strange circumstances of the therapy room, when the two are in love, the ethically correct action is to suspend the therapy and arrange for it to be continued by a colleague if necessary.

Cardinal Elements in Training

Theoretical learning, supervised clinical practice and personal therapy are the cardinal elements in training. It is difficult to discuss one without making an artificial distinction from the others as the three are so interrelated. Thus the section on each should be read with the others in mind. The reader is also invited to refer back to the section on what the individual therapist has to learn. The order of discussion reflects my priority. Many analytic therapists might wish to give primacy to personal therapy; many cognitive–behaviourists might dispute its relevance to their work. Academic courses awarding certificates, diplomas and masters are likely to emphasise theory and research. Many of the points made here are also relevant to training in other modalities of psychotherapy, such as group therapy (see Chapter 13).

Theoretical learning

Purpose and content

The purpose of training is to facilitate the exercise of natural abilities and acquired skills. To do this therapists need to gain extensive experience in the type(s) of therapy required for their practice, and for which affinity has been shown – in this case individual therapy. But to begin with, a conceptual framework of what therapy is about, how people mature and learn, and the role of the therapist is necessary. Later in training, theory will be critically examined to discover its areas of greater applicability and limitations. Studying theory means that therapists do not reinvent the wheel.

Learning theory is part of a broad educational process in which, in enlightened training, the development of informed, critical thinking is encouraged. Theory tends to be taught in an approach-specific way but general, overlapping and complementary perspectives also ought to be studied. Both specific and general learning need to be presented in the quantity and level appropriate to the trainee's need and ability. Ideally, theoretical learning would encompass the following:

1. *Theory and techniques specific to the therapy approach being learnt*
    In most trainings, this is the major component but, as has been indi-
    cated, the well-educated therapist needs to consider other aspects.

2. *The common therapeutic factors* Frank (1973) has argued
    strongly that in all effective therapies six influential factors are
    operative. The therapy (1) provides an exploratory rationale and
    (2) facilitates the exploration of traumas and conflictual issues in a
    state of emotional arousal. The effect is strengthened (3) when the
    therapist is sanctioned as a healer by the society. Responding to
    the patient's request for help (4) encourages that person to be
    hopeful about himself, and counters the demoralisation which
    typifies most patients' state. Therapy provides or prompts (5) suc-
    cess experiences. Finally, psychotherapy provides (6) an intense
    confiding relationship with a helping person. These factors have a
    much greater influence on outcome than the contribution made
    by approach-specific theory and technique (Lambert, 1986).

3. *The necessary conditions* Rogers (1957) proposed research stud-
    ies to support his proposition that three therapist conditions were
    necessary and sufficient for personality change: genuineness, un-
    conditional positive regard and accurate empathy. That these con-
    ditions are sufficient in themselves, are always helpful, and should
    be taken as absolutes has been much investigated and caveats
    placed on the original proposition. However, a sufficiency of each
    constitutes the basis of a helpful relationship. In passing, it should
    be noted that Freud took it as read that the analyst would be a
    decent, understanding, non-judgemental, respectful and neutral
    person. These qualities formed the basis of the therapeutic
    alliance and gave, in Ferenczi's words, stability (*Tragfestigheit*) to
    the relationship (Strupp, 1977).

4. *The evolution of psychotherapy ideas* How the concepts of psy-
    choanalysis, analytic psychology, individual psychology, existen-
    tialism, humanism, gestalt psychology, psychodrama, learning and
    systems theory have developed, their interrelationship and the
    implications for practice. In the analytic tradition, how an instinct-
    based theory has evolved to ego-psychology and then to self-
    psychology with the increasing emphasis on object-relations
    (human relations) and, especially in North America, on cultural
    and interpersonal aspects.

5. *Human development* How individuals develop over the life-
    span, with particular reference to maturational tasks, attachment
    theory, and the elements that contribute to being able, in Freud's
    definition of maturity, to love and to work.

6. *Mental mechanisms, character structure and the concept of
    conflict* How to make a dynamic formulation of the origin and

meaning of the patient's problems. The meaning and significance in clinical practice of the technical terms process, content,
therapeutic alliance, transference, countertransference and resistance. When and how to make effective interpretations and
other interventions. Good examples of the practical application
of these concepts may be found in Malan (1979) and Casement
(1985).

7. *Learning and systems theory* The role of shaping, modelling,
    generalisation and in vivo learning, and cognitions in determining
    human behaviour. The importance of problem definition and be-
    havioural analysis in making a diagnostic assessment. How be-
    havioural, system and dynamic processes operate in marriage and
    in families, and result in disturbed functioning. The contribution
    of psychological theory on cognitive dissonance, attribution theo-
    ry and crisis theory to the understanding of change and resistance
    to change.

8. *Ways in which therapists need to take account of linguistics,
    philosophy, religion and ethics in formulating a comprehensive
    model of human aspirations and functioning.*

9. *Cultural relativity with special reference to race, gender and age*
    The specific contribution made to twentieth-century understanding
    of role relationships and psychology by feminist psychology.

10. *Physical disease presenting as psychological disorder* Also the
    trainee will need to know the signs and symptoms of major psy-
    chiatric illness, the likely benefits and side-effects of psychotropic
    medication, and when and to whom to refer on. As a counterpart
    to this medical knowledge, the ways in which the sociological
    concepts of stigma and labelling further our understanding of al-
    ienation and isolation.

11. *Indications and contraindications for different kinds of
    therapies.*

12. *The vital role of support in therapy.*

13. *Preparation for therapy and patient–therapist matching* How
    negative effects arise through therapy and may be minimised.

14. *Research methodology and classic studies* How to evaluate the
    research literature and derive implications for clinical practice.

Format

Theory orders the great mass of clinical information and helps orientate
the therapist in finding a way forward. This useful function should not
curtail curiosity and the spirit of enquiry that is necessary for the development of the professional and the profession. Theory should
always be relevant and, depending on the level at which the training is
pitched, comprehensive in coverage.

How theory is presented varies greatly. Commonly the span of knowledge to be studied is set by the training organisers, a stance that has the virtue of making it clear what is to be learnt. Then there may be set readings, either by author or topic, an approach which specifies the route of study and makes it easy for trainer or trainee to spot omissions. However, it may have the negative effect of not engaging the student's active participation. An alternative, as in the South Trent training in dynamic psychotherapy with which I am involved, is to have a planning event each year where the trainees and seminar leaders jointly decide what is to be studied and how this is to be done. Instead of the conventional study of topics and authors, the question may be posed: What do I need to know in order to understand a specified psychotherapy process or problem? This is the approach of researching into a topic rather than simply reading someone else's selection of what is relevant. At the advanced level when many topics will have to be studied, teacher enthusiasm may be retained by offering a menu of courses in the teachers' areas of expertise which may be selected from by the trainee, with the training committee having the responsibility of ensuring that a balanced choice has been made.

Theory is not just to be found in textbooks. Novels, plays, films and poems portray the human condition more vividly, complexly and, often, more sensitively than do dry texts. Biographies and autobiographies trace individual lives (Holmes, 1986). All these should be studied.

Whatever the format, the trainee should return again and again to the fundamental, practical question: What are the implications of this theory or portrayal of life for *my* practice in *my* working environment with the patients that I see?

Supervised clinical practice

Clinical practice

Appropriate supervised practice is the central learning experience in training. The trainee needs to come to know what can be achieved in brief or focal work (8–25 weekly sessions), medium (40–70 sessions) and long-term therapy (upwards of 2–3 years). Weekly therapy is the most common mode in NHS psychotherapy and in many other settings; this has its own rhythm and intensity and is quite different from more frequent therapy, whose intensity may accelerate the process of change or be necessary in order to contain major personal disturbance. Weekly therapy tends to be more reality-oriented; two, three or five times a week therapy affords greater scope for exploration and regression. The two ends of the spectrum present different learning experiences and need to be sampled.

The supervisor has a key role in ensuring that patients with a wide range of problems and character structure are seen during the training period. Both breadth and depth of experience are important for the development of trainees. Breadth develops flexibility and highlights to the trainee problematic countertransferences and personal limitations that need either to be addressed in supervision, further experience and personal therapy, or avoided. Depth fosters stamina, the ability to contain intense feelings and to have the patience to move at the pace of someone whose sense of basic trust and confident autonomy is poorly developed; often this will mean enduring feeling powerless and helpless as the reality of the patient's inner world is engaged (Adler, 1972).

The same principle of breadth and depth in practice applies to supervision. To gain alternative perspectives against which the trainee's own view may develop, several supervisors need to be worked with for a year at a time. In order for the trainee to know one perspective in depth and to feel safe enough to explore certain doubts and conflicts, one main supervisor needs to be engaged with over 2 or 3 years. The choice of main supervisor is clearly a matter of great import.

What is judged to be an adequate training in terms of duration, frequency and amount of clinical practice varies between the psychotherapies. At the level of career psychotherapy, it is hard to see that fewer than 1000 hours of face-to-face individual therapy over 3–4 years at a rate of not less than 8 hours a week plus 325 hours of supervision divided between one main and two subsidiary supervisors could be sufficient, and this would need to be built on a foundation of less intensive, preliminary training in psychotherapy over 2 or more years.

In addition, trainees who are not qualified in one of the core mental health care professions need to gain through clinical placements sufficient acquaintance with major psychiatric illnesses in order to be able to recognise their presence; knowledge of the effects and likely benefits of pharmacological and physical treatment is also necessary. One example of why therapists need to be familiar with such matters is the high risk of suicide and depressive homicide in severe depressive illness; in such cases, antidepressants or ECT can be life-saving measures which restore normal functioning. Psychotherapists should not persist in interpreting psychopathology when a speedier and more effective biological remedy is at hand (Aveline, 1988). When patients are once more accessible to verbal interaction, and the risk of harm to themselves and their families has receded, then the precipitants and psychological vulnerabilities can be explored in psychotherapy, with the benefit of increased self-understanding and reduced likelihood of recurrence.

The role of the supervisor

The supervisor has a privileged, responsible position of mentor, guide and, often, assessor. From the advantageous position of hearing about therapy at second hand and generally after the event, the supervisor places his or her accumulated experience and knowledge at the service of the trainee. He or she helps the trainee work out with the patient the meaning and significance of the patient's communications, the nature of the patient's conflicts and, certainly in the more dynamic therapies, brings into sharp focus the way in which patient and therapist engage and how this may be turned to good account. In the beginning, the trainee will feel an ambivalent mixture of excitement and dread in taking on a new role. During this time of insecurity, and fearing being inadequate, he or she will need the support of the supervisor. As training progresses, the supervisor has to encourage the trainee to let go of the early, perhaps necessary, idealisation of the supervisor, so that identification can be replaced by an internalisation of professional skills (Gosling, 1978). In successful trainings, the trainee moves through the stages of inception, skills development and consolidation to mutuality of expertise with the trainer (Hess, 1986).

When patient and therapist concur in their appreciation of the aims of therapy, and also there is clarity in understanding accurately the structure of the conflicts and the process of the session, two major contributions have been made to the success of the endeavour. Many psychotherapy centres use a pre-assessment interview questionnaire to help clarify the purpose of the therapy; in Nottingham, this has questions on what the problems are, how people think they have come about and in what ways they have been shaped in their life, their self-concept, the characteristic form of their relationships, and what has prompted them to seek help now. Of course, in cognitive–behaviour therapy, goal-definition and objectification of problem severity as a baseline for therapy is an integral part of the approach. In whatever type of individual therapy, a formulation of the underlying dynamics is beneficial and, I would argue, necessary. Though different approaches will use their own vocabulary, schemata for the content are to be found in Aveline (1980), Cleghorn, Bellissimo and Will (1983), Perry, Cooper and Michels (1987) and Friedman and Lister (1987). I now favour an interpersonal formula which, in Strupp and Binder's (1984) approach, identifies a personally characteristic, recurrent narrative of acts of self, expectations of others, acts of others and introjects; though derived from analytic and cognitive approaches, the formula is atheoretical and may be used by all.

Whichever conceptual schema is used, the supervisor helps the supervisee to make fuller use of the session and, crucially in my view, to see how he or she is getting caught up in the self-limiting relationship patterns of the patient. Getting caught up is inevitable; the skill in psychotherapy is in recognising what is happening and using it constructively

(Aveline, 1989). In the phenomenon called 'negative fit', therapists act in ways that fit the patient's negative preconceptions which have been formed by how important people in his past would have responded to him. Thus, L. Luborsky and B. Singer (1974, unpublished data) demonstrated two major patterns of negative fit when the tape-recordings of experienced therapists were studied. One pattern was confirming the patient's fear of rejection by being critical, disapproving, cold, detached and indifferent, and the other was confirming the patient's fear of being made weak by being too directive, controlling and domineering. Clearly, every effort should be made in supervision to identify these two patterns and to turn the potentially negative impact to therapeutic effect. Often the supervisor will be able to guide the trainee in selecting suitable patients for the particular stage in training. In this situation, the supervisor may consider selecting pairings that promise well, as when the therapist has resolved in his or her life a similar conflict to the patient's, or avoiding pairings where the therapist seems likely only to reinforce the patient's pattern (see Chapter 4).

Ways of supervising

Pedder (1986) sees supervision in three ways: as being analogous to gardening, that is, as a process of promoting growth; as a place for play in the Winnicottian sense; and as being like therapy in that it provides a regular time and place for taking a second look at what happened in the therapy session. (Winnicott derived many of his ideas from his work with children. He saw psychotherapy taking place in the overlap of two playing areas, that of the patient and that of the therapist. The therapist's job is to help the patient move from a state of not being able to play into one of being able to play. Playing is a specially creative, intensely real activity which allows new syntheses to emerge.) Supervision aims to bring to the fore the creative potential of the therapist. It should be noted that supervision is not the same as therapy, though at times the distinction may become blurred.

Broadly speaking, the focus of supervisory interest can be on one of three areas: the process and content of the patient's concerns and communications; transference and countertransference reactions between therapist and patient; and the trainee–supervisor relationship. The focus on the last is justified by Doehrman's (1976) classic study which demonstrated the recreation in the trainer–supervisor relationship of the dynamics between patient and therapist and, at least theoretically, supports the view that, if the dynamics in supervision can be comprehended and resolved, blocks in the therapy relationship will be undone (for an example, see Caligor, 1984). In practice all these foci are useful, although in my practice, I incline towards the first as it is the patient's life that is my primary concern.

Much debate rages in psychotherapy circles about how the supervisory material should be presented. Classically in psychoanalytic training, a free-flowing account of the session is given, with much attention being paid to what is said and not said and the elucidation of countertransferences and associations as ways of illuminating unconscious processes. This is listening with the third ear (Reik, 1949). That the report may factually correspond poorly to the observable events of the session is held to be of little importance; indeed some supervisors argue that factually precise reporting both misses the point and may positively obscure it. I cannot accept this position. All ways of capturing the facts and essence of what went on are useful. Aids to supervision are just that – servants, not masters. They can be adapted to meet the needs of the moment.

After each session, trainees will write notes, detailing content, process and feeling issues. It is advantageous to have audio or video-recordings of the session, which may be viewed from the beginning or at a point of difficulty or interest or . . . not at all. Such recordings document the actual sequence of events and bring the dimensions of non-verbal and paralinguistic communication and change in emotional tone into the arena of supervision. Other means may be utilised. Transcripts allow the leisurely study of process and form of verbal interventions; as a semi-research exercise, the method of brief structured recall (Elliott and Shapiro, 1988) may be used to go over with the patient what were the most significant events in a session; the significant events are identified by the patient immediately after the session, then therapist and patient listen to the tape just before, during and after the event, and amplify through discussion the associated feelings, meaning and impact of that segment of interaction. Live supervision from behind a screen with either telephone contact or a 'bug in the ear' may also be employed, though such measures reduce the scope for the therapist to grapple alone with the patient's issues. There is more to be said for the supervisor leading the way in openness by occasionally putting his or her own tapes forward for discussion.

Being supervised is supposed to be helpful, but it can be persecutory (Bruzzone et al., 1985) and intrusive (Betcher and Zinberg, 1988). The trainer's self-esteem is vulnerable; there needs to be room in the training for privacy and for mistakes to be able to be made and discussed without dire penalty or excessive shame. Countertransference reactions on the part of the supervisor must not be forgotten. The trainee may represent the coming generation, who may equal or overtake the supervisor in skill and knowledge. Rivalry and the struggle for power may constitute a subtext for the supervisory meetings and, if not resolved, prove detrimental to professional development. A forum for supervisors to discuss problems in supervision is beneficial. In the training, it is also sensible and desirable in its own right to have group supervision as well as individual supervision, as the former provides multiple perspectives, peer support and the morale-enhancing opportunity of being of assistance to colleagues.

Skills development

While I favour weekly supervision over months and years as the best complement to the work of individual therapy, workshops and role-plays quickly lead to the acquisition of fundamental skills. Without risking any harm to the patient, difficult situations that therapists commonly face can be practised, the effects of different interventions observed and the model presented by more experienced therapists evaluated. Microcounselling training courses, first described at the end of the 1960s, have retained their promise for the relatively inexperienced trainee; they provide structured, focused learning over periods of 1, 2 or 3 days, with a strong emphasis on skills acquisition through role-play. At the more advanced approach-specific level, the use of detailed treatment manuals for such diverse approaches as supportive–expressive psychoanalytic psychotherapy, cognitive and interpersonal therapy of depression and short-term therapy is an interesting, effective, new method of skill development (Matarazzo and Patterson, 1986).

Personal therapy

'The therapist can only go as far with the patient as he can go himself', so the maxim runs. What therapists can find in themselves, they can recognise in others. Thus in addition to the resistance made by patients to dismantling defensive, outmoded, but originally adaptive, patterns, therapists contribute a resistance of their own to free exploration. The therapist's resistance may take the form of avoidance or over-interest; the former limits the opening up of areas of concern for the patient, the latter diverts the focus of the discourse to the therapist's own conflictual issues; these processes largely take place out of consciousness. Examples have been given in the sections on countertransference and the abuse of power, of some common personal conflicts which may limit or adversely distort the engagement of the therapist. All therapies at some stage confront reflective therapists with the dilemmas in their own lives and the partial solutions that they have adopted. An overlap of conflictual issue between therapist and patient often results in a blocked therapy, but may generate a particularly fruitful dyad when the therapist's conflict is not too great and the overlap enhances empathic contact.

Life experience and the practice of psychotherapy educate therapists about themselves. Self-scrutiny takes the learning about conflicts and

their resolution one step further, but the therapist's own internal security measures operate to maintain blind spots and protect self-esteem
from sobering self-realisations; these defences limit what can be done
alone. Personal therapy offers the therapist the same opportunity as the
patient has to explore, understand and resolve inner conflicts. It brings
together theoretical learning and psychotherapy practice in an experience that makes personal sense of the two. At a practical level, personal
therapy provides a means through which sufficient self-understanding
can be gained for therapists to recognise how their personality and life
experience affect their ability to be objective, and to reduce their tendency to impose their own solutions on the life problems of their
patients (Joint Committee on Higher Psychiatric Training, 1987). The
nature of the conflicts that interfere with therapists' work predicate
their requirements for therapy in terms of type, duration and frequency, and the achievement of sufficient resolution in order to work
more effectively indicates the end-point of personal therapy on the
practical level. At the next level, therapy aims to enhance therapists'
abilities to relate, empathically and creatively, to their patients. One
element in this is knowing at first hand what it is like to be a patient;
another is the loosening through therapy of the self-limiting grip of
personal conflicts. Beyond that, as was detailed in the section on
motivating factors in the therapist, therapy offers an opportunity for
therapists to heal themselves, an unmet need which may have been of
prime importance in the selection by the trainee therapist of this kind
of work. At a sociological level, personal therapy has the function of a
rite of passage, forming and affirming their identity as a psychotherapist and as a member of their professional group.

Perhaps the most compelling argument in favour of personal therapy
is that every therapist, like every patient, sees the world through the
perspective of their guiding fictions, and is impelled to impose that
order and those patterns on others. Thus the more therapists are aware
of what are their personal, determining fictions, the more likely they
will be able to engage with the reality of the other.

Personal therapy in varying intensity and duration is a required component of most formal, advanced trainings in psychotherapy; in psychoanalysis, full personal analysis is mandatory. In psychoanalysis, the
sequence of engagement in training is being in therapy, then theory
seminars, and finally conducting analyses. In Henry's (1977) survey of
4000 North American psychotherapists, 74 per cent had been in personal therapy and nearly 50 per cent had re-entered therapy for two to
four periods; conversely, 36 per cent had chosen not to pursue that
course. Despite the consensus in favour of personal therapy, especially
at the psychodynamic end of the spectrum, there is little published
evidence of its efficacy in enhancing therapeutic ability. Surveys of the

literature by Greenberg and Staller (1981) and Macaskill (1988) conclude that first, 15–33 per cent of trainees have unsatisfactory personal
therapy experiences, e.g. damage to marriage, destructive acting-out
and excessive withdrawal from the outside world; second, therapy
early in the therapist's career may have deleterious effects on work
with patients; and third, there is no positive correlation between either
the fact of having been in therapy or its duration on the outcome of the
therapist's professional work. The level of reported dissatisfaction is in
line with that generally expected for negative effects in psychotherapy,
and, as such, emphasises the importance of the trainee making a sage
choice of therapist.

When personal therapy is decided upon, its intensity and duration
should parallel the form of psychotherapy that the therapist is going to
practise. Generally, this will be one or more times a week for 3 or more
years. It is important that the therapist enters therapy not only because
the training requires it, but also to resolve personal conflicts or difficulties that are being encountered in his or her work and life. Advice on
whom to consult should be sought from an experienced adviser who
can steer the trainee away from pairings that are less than optimal, and
towards those of greater promise (Coltart, 1987). Exploratory sessions
should be held with several potential therapists before the choice is
made. This counsel of perfection could well apply to patients if ever
they were in the position of being able to choose whom to see.

Evaluation

During training, there should be opportunities for evaluation, both for-
matively and normatively. It will be recalled that, in educational terms,
'formative' evaluation refers to non-examined elements that enrich the
educational experience of training, whereas 'normative' refers to entry/
exit, pass/fail criteria. The aims of the training should be clearly stated
and be attainable within the learning experiences of the scheme. A system for monitoring progress both by self-assessment and by the trainers
is necessary, as is the giving of feedback so as to help trainees improve
the quality of their psychotherapy. Individual and psychometric assessment of severity of patient problem can form a baseline for the evaluation of the success of therapy. Case books recording progress and any
alteration in formulation document the range of therapy experience and
the lessons to be learnt, not from books but from actual practice. Detailed written case accounts of one or more psychotherapies carried out
by the trainee demonstrate the degree of the trainee's development and
bring into focus how difficulties have been encountered and struggled
with. Personal tutors have a key role as adviser and appraiser to trainees
finding their way through the training. Ultimately, evaluation should

address the question of therapist competence: how effective is this therapist in aiding the quest of his or her patients towards more fruitful living?
The methodology to assess this does not yet exist. Only partial progress
has been made towards the subsidiary but important question of what
this training has added to the therapist's ability; one example is the
quantification of the improvement in interviewing skills acquired
through microcounselling courses (Matarazzo and Patterson, 1986).

Supportive Psychotherapy

The rhetoric of psychotherapy is towards fundamental change in
people's feelings, attitudes and interactions; this has been the type of
individual therapy for which training has been described in this chapter. The trainee therapist in his or her enthusiasm and inexperience of
the struggle to survive that many patients face may be tempted to press
for a pace and depth of change for which the patient is not ready.
Fundamental change will not be possible or desirable for all or, if possible, no authorisation may be given by the patient for deep exploration
which may profoundly challenge his or her view of him- or herself. This
situation has to be explicitly respected and the value of support recognised and taught in training. All therapy has to have in it a sufficiently
supportive element in order to help the patient contend with the up-
heaval of change: most therapies will move between challenging and
supportive phases. Furthermore, supportive psychotherapy is a subject
in its own right. It is indicated for the many individuals who need
sustained support in order to return them to their optimal level of
adjustment and maintain them here. It has its own complex skills and
needs to be learnt by even the most therapeutically ambitious therapist.

Registration

At present, anyone in Britain may practise as a psychotherapist and
advertise their services as such. Unlike North America and many Euro-
pean countries, psychotherapy is not a regulated profession. No formal
training or subscription to a code of ethics is required. Within institutions such as the NHS, universities and polytechnics, the consumer of
psychotherapy has the protection of knowing that for the most part the
therapist will have been appointed in open competition with other
applicants, and has the sanction of being able to initiate an official
complaint. Membership of professions that are regulated by statutory
bodies as, for example, is medicine by the General Medical Council, or
of training institutes with regulatory powers, affords some assurance
that the standards of the therapist are adequate and will be maintained.

But in the private sector, members of the public have little protection against the misinformed or unethical therapist. This is bad for the consumer and bad for the profession.

The Foster Report (1971), a Government-appointed enquiry, recommended that the profession of psychotherapy be regulated by statute. Seven years later, the Sieghart Report (1978) proposed the establishment of a council which would draw up and enforce a code of professional ethics and approve training courses. Registration of individuals as psychotherapists would be indicative rather than functional, that is, on the basis of titles associated with various forms of psychotherapy. The desirable goal of registration as some guarantee of integrity and competence has since not made much progress. A Private Member's Bill in Parliament failed and the core professions have not been able to agree on a common position. For several years, a talking shop of psychotherapy organisations has been held each year in Rugby (the Rugby Conference), initially under the auspices of the British Association for Counselling. The participating organisations have with some difficulty grouped into six sections: analyst, analytical, behavioural, family/marital/sexual, and humanistic and integrative psychotherapy plus hypnotherapy and neurolinguistic programming. In 1989 the conference adopted a formal constitution. It is possible that this body may become *de facto* a registering body. Whether this occurs or not, some form of registration and, for that matter, re-registration is likely to come into being.

Implicit in the above is the proposition that continued attention to competence is part of the professional attitude of the psychotherapist. This is particularly important for the individual therapist, as that person tends to work in relative or absolute isolation and, in the absence of challenging opportunities for further learning, may develop poor working practices. Feedback from colleagues in peer-group supervision of actual clinical work is especially helpful.

Conclusion

The current practice of psychotherapy distils out what is known about human healing. In its practice it is both an art and a science: both elements need to be borne in mind in training. Training may occur in phases but is a lifelong commitment. Competence is achievable, but there is always more for the therapist to learn. No end-point has been reached in the development of individual therapy as an agent of personal change. Further refinement in theory, scope and practice can be expected, especially if the practitioners of the different individual psychotherapies learn to speak with one another in pursuit of the common goal of assisting patients to lead more fruitful lives.

References

ADLER, G. (1972). Helplessness in the helpers. *British Journal of Medical Psychology* **45**, 315–325.

AUERBACH, A.A. and JOHNSON, M. (1977). Research on the therapist's level of experience. In: A.S. Gurman and A.M. Razin (Eds) *Effective Psychotherapy*. Oxford: Pergamon Press.

AVELINE, M.O. (1980). Making a psychodynamic formulation. *Bulletin of the Royal College of Psychiatrists* **4**, 192–193.

AVELINE, M.O. (1986). The corrective emotional experience, a fundamental unifying concept in psychotherapy. Paper presented at the Annual Conference of the Society for Psychotherapy Research, Wellseley College, Massachusetts, June.

AVELINE, M.O. (1988). The relationship of drug therapy and psychotherapy. *Current Opinion in Psychiatry,* **1**, 309–313.

AVELINE, M.O. (1989). The provision of illusion in psychotherapy. *Midland Journal of Psychotherapy* **1**, 9–16.

BENNET, G. (1987). *The Wound and the Doctor*. London: Secker & Warburg.

BERNSTEIN, L. and BERNSTEIN, R.S. (1980). *Interviewing: A Guide for Health Professionals*. New York: Appleton-Century-Crofts.

BETCHER, R.W. and ZINBERG, N.E. (1988). Supervision and privacy in psychotherapy training. *American Journal of Psychiatry* **145**, 796–803.

BRUZZONE, M., CASAULA, E., JIMENZ, J.P. and JORDAN, J.F. (1985). Regression and persecution in analytic training: reflections on experience. *International Review of Psycho-Analysis* **12**, 411–415.

BUGENTAL, J.F.T. (1964). The person who is the psychotherapist. *Journal of Counseling Psychology* **28**, 272–277.

BURTON, A. (1975). Therapist satisfaction. *American Journal of Psychoanalysis* **35**, 115–122.

CALIGOR, L. (1984). Parallel and reciprocal processes in psychoanalytic supervision. In: L. Caligor, P.M. Bromberg and J.D. Meltzer (Eds) *Clinical Perspectives on the Supervision of Psychoanalysis and Psychotherapy*. New York: Plenum Press.

CASEMENT, P. (1985). *On Learning from the Patient*. London: Tavistock.

CLEGHORN, J.M., BELLISIMO, A. and WILL, D. (1983). Teaching some principles of individual psychodynamics through an introductory guide to formulations. *Canadian Journal of Psychiatry* **28**, 162–172.

COLTART, N. (1987). Diagnosis and assessment for suitability for psycho-analytical psychotherapy. *British Journal of Psychotherapy* **4**, 127–134.

DAVIS, J.D., ELLIOTT, R., DAVIS, M.L., BINNS, M., FRANCIS, V.M., KELMAN, J.E. and SCHRODER, T.A. (1987). Development of a taxonomy of therapist difficulties: initial report. *British Journal of Medical Psychology* **60**, 109–119.

DOEHRMAN, M.J.G. (1976). Parallel processes in supervision and psychotherapy. *Bulletin of the Menninger Clinic* **40**, 1–104.

ELLIOTT, R. and SHAPIRO, D.A. (1988). Brief structured recall: a more efficient method for studying significant therapy moments. *British Journal of Medical Psychology* **61**, 141–153.

FAIRBAIRN, W.R.D. (1954). *An Object-Relations Theory of the Personality*. New York: Basic Books.

FARBER, B.A. (1983). The effects of psychotherapeutic practice upon psychotherapists. *Psychotherapy: Theory, Research and Practice* **20**, 174–182.

FARBER, B.A. and HEIFETZ, L.J. (1981). The satisfactions and stresses of psychotherapy work: a factor analytic study. *Professional Psychology* **12**, 621–630.

FLEMING, J. (1987). *The Teaching and Learning of Psychoanalysis*. New York: Guilford Press.

FOSTER, J.G. (1971). *Enquiry into the Practice and Effects of Scientology*. London: HMSO.

FRANK, J.D. (1973). *Persuasion and Healing*, 2nd edn. New York: Schocken Books.

FRIEDMAN, R.S. and LISTER, P. (1987). The current status of the psychodynamic formulation. *Psychiatry* **50**, 126–141.

GOSLING, R. (1978). Internalization of the trainer's behaviour in professional training. *British Journal of Medical Psychology* **51**, 35–40.

GREBEN, S.E. (1975). Some difficulties and satisfactions inherent in the practice of psychoanalysis. *International Journal of Psycho-Analysis* **56**, 427–433.

GREBEN, S.E. (1984). *Love's Labor*. New York: Schocken Books.

GREENBERG, R.P. and STALLER, J. (1981). Personal therapy for therapists. *American Journal of Psychiatry* **138**, 1, 467–471.

GREENSON, R.R. (1967). *The Technique and Practice of Psychoanalysis*, vol. 1. New York: International Universities Press.

GUGGENBUHL-CRAIG, A. (1979). *Power in the Helping Profession*. Irving, TX: Spring Publications.

GUY, J.D. (1987). *The Personal Life of the Psychotherapist*. New York: Wiley.

HEIMANN, P. (1950). On counter-transference. *International Journal of Psychoanalysis* **31**, 81–84.

HENRY, W.A. (1977). Personal and social identities of psychotherapist. In: A.S. Gurman and A.M. Razin (Eds) *Effective Psychotherapy*. Oxford: Pergamon Press.

HESS, A.K. (1986). Growth in supervision: stages of supervisee and supervisor development. In: F.W. Kaslow (Ed) *Supervision and Training: Models, Dilemmas, Challenges*. New York: Haworth Press.

HOLMES, J. (1986). Teaching the psychotherapeutic method: some literary parallels. *British Journal of Medical Psychology* **59**, 113–121.

HOLROYD, J.C. and BRODSKY, A.M. (1977). Psychologists' attitudes and practices regarding erotic and non-erotic physical contact with patients. *American Psychologist* **32**, 843–849.

JOINT COMMITTEE ON HIGHER PSYCHIATRIC TRAINING (1987). *Requirements for Specialist Training in Psychotherapy*. London: Royal College of Psychiatriasts.

JONES, E. (1913). The God complex. *Essays in Applied Psychoanalysis*, vol. 2. London: Hogarth Press.

LAMBERT, M.J. (1986). Implications of psychotherapy outcome research for eclectic psychotherapy. In: J.C. Norcross (Ed.) *Handbook of Eclectic Psychotherapy*. New York: Brunner Mazel.

LOMAS, P. (1981). *The Case for a Personal Psychotherapy*. Oxford: Oxford University Press.

LUBORSKY, L., SINGER, B. and LUBORSKY, L. (1975). Comparative studies of psychotherapies: is it true that 'Everyone has won and all must have prizes?'. *Archives of General Psychiatry* **32**, 995–1008.

MACASKILL, N.D. (1988). Personal therapy in the training of the psychotherapist: is it effective? *British Journal of Psychotherapy* **4**, 219–226.

MALAN, D. (1979). *Individual Psychotherapy and the Science of Psychodynamics*. London: Butterworths.

MARMOR, J. (1953). The feeling of superiority: an occupational hazard in the practice of psychotherapy. *American Journal of Psychiatry* **110**, 370–373.

MARMOR, J. (1972). Sexual acting-out in psychotherapy. *American Journal of Psycho-Analysis* **22**, 3–8.

MATARAZZO, R.G. and PATTERSON, D.R. (1986). Methods of teaching therapeutic skill. In: S.L. Garfield and A.L. Bergin (Eds) *Handbook of Psychotherapy and Behavior Change*, 3rd edn. New York: Wiley.

MENNINGER, K. (1958). *Theory of Psychoanalytic Technique*. New York: Basic Books.

PEDDER, J. (1986). Reflections on the theory and practice of supervision. *Psycho-analytic Psychotherapy* 2, 1–12.

PERRY, S., COOPER, A.M. and MICHELS, R. (1987). The psychodynamic formulation: its purpose, structure, and clinical application. *American Journal of Psychiatry* 144, 543–550.

REIK, T. (1949). *Listening with the Third Ear*. New York: Farrer, Straus.

ROGERS, C.R. (1957). The necessary and sufficient conditions of therapeutic person-ality change. *Journal of Consulting Psychology* 21, 95–103.

ROSIN, S.A. and KNUDSON, R.M. (1986). Perceived influence of life experiences on clinical psychologists' selection and development of theoretical orientations. *Psychotherapy* 23, 357–363.

SANDLER, J. (1988). Psychoanalysis and psychoanalytic psychotherapy: problems of differentiation. Paper read at Conference on Psychoanalysis and Psychoanalytic Psychotherapy (Association of Psychoanalytic Psychotherapy in the NHS), Lon-don, 22–23 April 1988.

SCHAFER, R. (1983). *The Analytic Attitude*. London: Hogarth Press.

SIEGHART, P. (1978). *Statutory Registration of Psychotherapists*. London: Tavistock Clinic.

STORR, A. (1979). *The Art of Psychotherapy*. London: Secker & Warburg.

STRUPP, H.H. (1960). *Psychotherapists in Action*. New York: Grune & Stratton.

STRUPP, H.H. (1977). A reformulation of the dynamics of the therapist's contribution. In: A.S. Gurman and A.M. Razin (Eds) *Effective Psychotherapy*. Oxford: Pergamon Press.

STRUPP, H.H. and BINDER, J.L. (1984). *A Guide to Time-Limited Dynamic Psycho-therapy*. New York: Basic Books.

Chapter 12
The Use of Audio- and Video-tape Recordings of Therapy Sessions in the Supervision and Practice of Dynamic Psychotherapy

Introduction

Supervision is a cardinal element in training to practise dynamic psychotherapy, the other elements being theoretical learning and, in most if not all training schemes, personal therapy. The purpose of training is to facilitate the exercise of natural abilities and acquired skills to the best effect (see Chapter 11). The advent of easily made audio and video recordings of therapy sessions opens the way for such recordings to become essential aids in the supervision of individual dynamic psychotherapy (as they are already in behavioural and family psychotherapy); in addition, recordings constitute a resource which may be used with caution in therapy itself, and more straightforwardly, in research and clinical audit.

Recording provides direct, factually correct access to the therapy session which on that level cannot be matched by the common, indirect method in supervision of the supervisee giving a recollected and impressionistic account of what happened. Despite the many advantages of an electronic record, the indirect method is preferred by many psychoanalytic psychotherapists, and anything different is anathema to some. This paper suggests some reason for the preference. The advantages and disadvantages of recording are examined, as is the meaning for the patient of being recorded. Advice is given on

From M.O. Aveline (1990) 'Supervision as a way of learning', Workshop at the Second Tavistock Clinic Symposium on Supervision, London, 31 July–2 August 1990.

making recordings, ethical issues and confidentiality. Finally, other uses of recordings are considered.

The Direct Access–Indirect Recollection Controversy

A supervisor of dynamic psychotherapy may concentrate on one of three foci during the supervisory hour: the process and content of the patient's concerns and communciations, transference and counter-transference reactions between patient and therapist, and the supervisee–supervisor relationship as a mirror image of the psycho-dynamic relationship between patient and therapist. These foci are neither mutually exclusive nor absolute requirements for good super-vision, but they do identify dominant styles of supervision, each having the justification of custom and theory. Generalising, the more psycho-analytic the orientation of the supervisory pair, the more the super-vision will tend towards the second and third foci. My focus as an interpersonal psychotherapist is towards the first and second (see Chapter 15).

At the psychoanalytic end of the spectrum, the supervisee may place on one side the process notes about the sessions to be reported and give a free-flowing account with much emphasis on countertrans-ference feelings, evoked fantasies and mental associations. The uncon-scious processes of the patient, their meaning and engagement with the conscious and unconscious processes of the therapist are illumin-ated by the form in which the sessions are presented. What is not said by the supervisee in his account may be of equal significance with that which is said; omissions tell their own story, just as do fantasies, asso-ciations and countertransference feelings. It is to these phenomena that the supervisor attends; he listens with the third ear (Reik, 1949). In short, this style of supervision mimics the style of the psychoanalytic hour. Factually precise reporting is held not to be on the right level and may even obscure the better level. This is an important reason why the use of audio and video recordings is not supported by some supervisors.

The justification for the method of indirect recollection is rooted in psychoanalytic technique and theory. Freud (1912) advocated a par-ticular form of listening on the part of the clinician, that of ' "evenly suspended attention" in the face of all that one hears' . . . 'he should simply listen and not bother about whether he is keeping anything in mind' (pp. 111–112). The purpose is to avoid the 'perceptual falsifica-tion' which follows from the therapist being selective in which mater-ial he attends to: 'In making the selection if he follows his expectations, he is in danger of never finding anything but what he already knows.' In a similar vein, Bion (1967) enjoined the therapist to enter each session 'without memory and desire'. Putting to one side the debate about the feasibility or even the desirability of the therapist being without intentionality, the method of 'evenly suspended attention' with its neutrality as to focus allows the patient the utmost freedom in determining what he wants to talk about in therapy, and provides the therapist and, beyond him the supervisor, with a powerful tool for understanding the inner processes of the patient's mind through attending to the form of the relationship that the two have, first in the dyad of patient and therapist, and secondly that of supervisee and supervisor.

The focus on the dyad of supervisee and supervisor, which at first sight is far removed from the patient's concerns, received powerful reinforcement in Doehrman's (1976) classic study of psychoanalytic psychotherapy; she consolidated established practice. Doehrman demonstrated that the dynamic relationship between patient and therapist was recreated in the relationship that the therapist had with his supervisor, the 'parallel process'. Furthermore, the process was two-way: not only did the relationship of the patient with the therapist colour that with the supervisor, but the relationship of the supervisee and the supervisor was played out for better or worse with the patient. The progress of the patient was crucially dependent on how well the recreations were identified and worked with in the supervision (see also Caligor, 1984). In a series of only eight supervisor–therapist–patient trios, Doehrman documented a process that undoubtedly occurs and that may be addressed productively. However, as an empirical justification for making this *the* focus in supervision, the evidence is slight. No comparative studies have been made of effectiveness of therapy when this or either of the two other styles of supervision is deployed.

Other reasons why the use of audio and video recordings in supervision is controversial have to do with privacy, confidentiality and ethical considerations. Psychotherapists rightly guard the confidences to which they are privy, but may also have an emotional attachment to the idea of absolute privacy, and find comfort in the indirectness of reporting sessions through recollection. Then, despite the fact that process notes are a tangible record of the session and the privacy of the therapy hour is already compromised in the act of offering it for supervision, they may perceive the ideal as being destroyed by the recording. They may also feel that their valued position of neutrality is eroded by their introducing the recorder into the frame of therapy. Of course, the first task of the therapist is to foster the creation in therapy of a psychologically safe place wherein the patient may explore his difficulties. For some patients, it is unethical to ask permission to record sessions, either because of the detail of their concerns or because their fragility as people would be tested to breaking point by being recorded. This is an argument for being selective and sensitive, not an argument of general objection. These practical issues are considered later.

In teasing out some of the reasons for controversy, no argument is being made to replace traditional styles of supervision with the fruit of technology. Rather, the case is made for recordings as a supplementary source of information, with definite advantages and disadvantages, and which, subject to certain constraints, should be available to supervisee and supervisor (Wolberg, 1988).

Advantages and Disadvantages

The word supervision is derived from the Latin *super* meaning 'over' and *videre* 'to see'. In a literal sense, audio and video recordings provide a direct, factually correct vision of what transpired in the therapy session. It is this direct access, unfiltered through the therapist's recollections, that is the prime advantage of the recording. The patient and therapist can be heard in action, and seen if recorded on video, which is a very different matter from those events being reported. The simple exercise of comparing one's notes on a session with a tape-recording dramatically highlights the deficiencies of memory, especially when emotionally charged and complex issues are emerging and being explored. In recollection, whole segments of interaction are not recorded in memory, the sequence of interactions becomes reordered, key statements by the patient are either misheard or not heard, elements are magnified or diminished, and interpretations take on a wishful perfection.

Bromberg (1984), a declared supporter of the integrated use of audio-tapes, writes 'In supervision, the student must be able to scrutinise what he already does. He must have the opportunity to hear his sessions, to hear himself with his patient, in a way that goes beyond what he heard during the sessions as they were in progress' (p. 35). Just as the one-way screen in the early days of family therapy provided the supporting team with a relatively neutral view of the session, so do recordings enable the supervisor in a literal sense to hear and the supervisee to hear again his work (Cade and Cornwell, 1985). It is particularly valuable for therapists, at all levels of seniority, periodically to review in private tapes of their sessions, a form of professional self-audit (Rioch, Coulter and Weinberger, 1976).

As a supervisor, an audio or video recording, provided it is of sufficient quality, brings the patient alive and increases my involvement. The Socratic dictum 'Speak, in order that I may see you' holds. I am stimulated by the way in which words are used, the metaphors deployed and the images evoked. Snatches of interaction often vividly illustrate the central dilemmas of a person's life. Verbal, sub-verbal and non-verbal communication may be addressed. The medium is particularly well placed to identify such phenomena as the patient filling all the space of the session with words, so as to leave no room for the therapist to say anything for fear that what might be said will disrupt the inner equilibrium; the nervous laugh that as surely indicates that there is an issue of importance at hand as does the bird with a trailing wing that the nest is nearby; the therapist whose words of encouragement are belied by his impatient tone or gesture; and the patient whose placatory dependence is shot through with hostility. Wolberg (1988) gives a graphic example of a female patient with deepening depression and a history of having a busy mother and distant father. On the video-tape, it was seen that the therapist unconsciously recreated this depressing situation by placing his chair so that he faced *away* from her. The recording gives access to another layer of communication and meaning whose significance, once identified, can be explored. This level can certainly be addressed in the reportage of recollection but, without direct access to the session, more turns upon the skill of the supervisee in giving his account and the sensitivity of the supervisor to these subtle, important nuances of interaction.

Key moments can be played again and again for microanalysis. What was said? How was it said? What did it mean? How did the supervisee or other members of the supervisory group feel? What is going on? What does this say about the patient's problematic dynamics? In what ways are the relationship difficulties of the patient in everyday life being played out in the therapy relationship? What might happen next? How might one intervene and why? What actually happened? And so on . . . Technique may be studied, as may times of drama, breakthrough, success and failure.

A final advantage, though one of chance rather than election, is that the act of recording constitutes a powerful element in the gestalt of therapy, and may become another facet to be understood and worked with. All is grist to the therapeutic mill.

There are several significant disadvantages to recording. Recording always has an effect on therapy; its meaning needs to be explored (see below). It may be abusive to the patient. In the encounter of therapy, the patient is in a weak position, desperately seeking a remedy for his demoralisation and loss of mastery, and easily subject to an abuse of power by the therapist (Guggenbuhl-Craig, 1971; see Chapter 11). Voyeuristic and sadistic tendencies in the therapist and supervisor may be acted out in requiring the recording of intimate details which have been given in trust to one person, the therapist, but which will be reviewed in another setting with unknown people who have not been party to the confidence. Patients with a history of childhood sexual or physical abuse may find it hard enough to speak of their experience without the extra stress of being exposed to recording; for some, the experience in therapy may traumatically reverberate with the coercion of childhood. Paranoid patients, or those with so little trust that recording is unacceptable to them, may be precluded from therapy if taping is rigidly insisted upon. Conversely, exhibitionistic patients may be encouraged in their proclivity.

From the point of view of the therapist, taping may theoretically compromise his neutrality. A more cogent objection to taping is that it is oppressive to the therapist. Therapists need to develop their own creative way of doing therapy; they need to make mistakes and struggle to find solutions. A degree of privacy facilitates learning. Certainly doing therapy is an intensely personal activity, and confronts the thoughtful therapist with his strengths and limitations as a person. Playing a tape is nearly always stressful for the therapist, and a pattern of collusive avoidance often develops in supervision, the therapist sparing himself exposure and the feared attack of his overcritical super-ego and the supervisor identifying with the supervisee and being overprotective. How these issues are handled in supervision is a crucial determinant of whether or not the supervisee needs the cloak of privacy in order to develop his skills. Is the recording being used to humiliate the supervisee by highlighting deficiencies, or to aid collaborative work between colleagues and potential equals? The same dynamic can operate in supervisions based on recollection.

The argument against taping that it encourages having a focus in supervision, thus interfering with 'evenly suspended attention', and the wrong focus at that has already been rehearsed. Attending to microepisodes in a session may miss the larger dynamic processes that are more important, and distract the supervisory group from exploring them. It is held to be more valuable to approach the task of understanding the session on a poetic, intuitive level, rather than that of factual reality. These objections posit an either/or reality in supervision which, if it exists, reflects an elective choice made by the supervisor. All levels need to be considered. Taping is a supervisory aid; it is servant, not master.

The mechanical disadvantages should not be underestimated. Recording equipment is intrusive, takes time to set up, and often produces tapes with poor-quality sound and image. Finding the right moment on the tape is difficult and listening to any more than brief sequences is very time-consuming. The method contributes its own distortions; the impression of anger, for example, may be accentuated. In addition, for the supervisor and supervisory group, it is difficult to listen to intimate moments and distressing experiences without having earned the right to hear them through direct work with the patient; it stirs uncomfortable feelings of voyeurism and helplessness. Finally, it is difficult to guarantee the security of tapes.

The Use of Tapes in Supervision

Tapes lend themselves to many purposes. Three are discussed: trainees' tapes in supervision and in assessment of their development as therapists, and supervisor's tapes. In Nottingham, all trainee therapists audio-tape their sessions; video equipment is available. They write detailed process notes, often informed by listening to the tape. In my supervisions, the therapist gives an overview of the session(s) which prompts discussion and may or may not lead on to the tape being played, the latter being a common occurrence. The tape is there to be used flexibly and appropriately. The tape may be played from the beginning or from near the end, both being times when dynamic issues may be particularly clear. Alternatively, a special point of interest, identified by the trainee (with the tape already correctly positioned), fellow trainees in a group supervision, or the supervisor, is played. The choice of moment might be to illustrate what felt like a key interaction, a time when an intervention went well or badly, or the therapist felt stuck, or simply to listen with a prior discussion of the dynamics in mind to see what evidence of confirmation or disconfirmation accrues. Collegiate learning is promoted if the choice of when to play the tape and which moment is shared among all the participants in the supervision.

The chosen moment is played and replayed with a fuller hearing on each repetition. It would be unusual to play more than a few minutes, or even seconds, without some feeling, new thought or association being triggered and leading to discussion. Occasionally, 10–15 minutes might be played to hear how the session develops over a longer period, and to monitor the therapist's way of intervening and sense of timing. Special attention is paid to the process of the relationship, not just to content, and to alterations in tone and posture. Times of increased tension often signal the engagement of core conflicts and the opportunity for intervention and dynamic change (see Chapter 2). Technique may be examined, as may the significance of the discrepancies between the therapist's report and what is observed on the tape. Microanalysis, as described in the previous section, fosters the elaboration of alternative formulations, which may be tested by asking the group to make predictions as to what will happen next; the actual sequence may be followed and its consequences charted.

If tapes are kept, they give tangible evidence of the degree of change in both patient and therapist over time. Through comparing tapes, trainees may see how their formation as therapists is progressing, and identify areas of performance that need further work.

It is highly beneficial for the supervisor to play his tapes occasionally for supervision by the supervisees. Not only will the supervisor learn from the experience but any oppressive myth of the supervisor's great superiority in dealing with the issues of therapy will be dispelled, and the trainees will be encouraged to think for themselves and develop their own strengths. A model of openness and willingness to learn is being portrayed. So often in supervision, there is a hidden, destructive struggle betweem supervisor and supervisee to be 'one up', or avoid being 'one down'. This dynamic is undermined when the supervisor has the courage to show his own work (Rioch, 1980). Also, learning is advanced by seeing experienced therapists at work. An illustration can be worth a thousand words: suddenly a whole range of new possibilities is opened up. Seeing how some issue or dilemma is handled provides a model if the practice is good and, when less appealing, a point of comparison which prompts the viewer to affirm how and why his practice differs. Psychotherapists, being for the most part practical people, have their attention vividly engaged when material – that dry, dreadful word for what transpires in therapy – is presented. Finally, viewing a video-tape of a supervisory session, either alone or with other supervisors, is an excellent way for the necessary task of the supervisor to evaluate his style and performance in supervision (Fleming and Benedek, 1966).

The Meaning for the Patient of Being Taped

Being taped is never a neutral event for the patient. Its meaning is not fixed, but is often persecutory in tone. Therapy advances as trust-worthiness is demonstrated by the therapist and the patient's trust builds up. The recorder represents a tangible link into the outside work. Though the door into the consulting room is closed, a conduit is open. Confidentiality, so vital an element in therapy, is threatened. For this reason, it is good practice to have as part of the therapy agreement the provision that the patient can have the tape turned off at any moment that he does not want recorded. In practice, this right, once given, is rarely exercised. When tapes are used for supervision, it is important to emphasise to the patient that the recording is for the therapist's benefit, to advance his understanding and performance.

Just as with a one-way screen, the recorder readily becomes the object of projections. The listeners laugh at what they hear, they make humiliating and derogatory comments, they broadcast abroad the patient's secrets, and, worst of all, the therapist, so seemingly understanding in the session, betrays his true colours by joining in this assault when in possession of the tape and away from the session. These are extreme, common reactions which need to be addressed as they occur. They say much about the patient's inner world. Some patients find being taped too stressful, at least in the early stages of therapy. Their objection must be respected. Others use being recorded in a defensive way. If only the recorder was not there, then they would work, then they would disclose. This is resistance and, as such, needs to be worked with. Often significant communications will be reserved for when the recorder is not on; there may be a change of tone to a more intimate or less formal way of talking, a confidence given or a hidden anxiety revealed. The same phenomenon happens in non-taped sessions when the patient is on the threshold of the consulting room, either entering or, more commonly, leaving, and, as it were, can construe the moment as being outside the therapy hour, with a greater freedom to express what is important and potentially escape from exploration. These communications and their timing need to be considered in the enquiry of therapy.

Being taped may feel abusive to patients whose sense of personal mastery and proper boundaries has been attacked by coercion and abuse of power by powerful figures in their formative past. A woman, whose father had derided her views and regularly beaten her to try and induce her to submit to his control, was unable to refuse being taped for a teaching event. Though inwardly angry, she felt unable to protest for two reasons: first, the request felt like a hurdle that she had to jump lest she be seen to be not trying in therapy, and hence at risk of being abandoned and thrown out of therapy. Secondly, to disclose her inner turmoil was to be vulnerable and weak and would, she feared, lay herself open to abuse by the therapist when he sensed the power of his position. Were she to show her anger, she would never be able to return. Therefore, it was safer to accede and, secretly, be resentful. In the event, this recreation of a conflictual situation of central import-ance for her had a corrective resolution. Her clenched fists, buried in her coat pockets, told the untold story of her dilemma. As the situation was explored, she exploded with anger over the therapist daring to know what was best for her. Even more important therapeutically was that she was able to return the following week and maintain a good relationship with the therapist; she reported feeling liberated in her interactions during the week.

Reactions are not always persecutory. The tape may symbolise the therapist's interest and concern. When a session is not recorded, it may be taken to mean loss of interest, that the patient is boring or beyond help, and that discharge is imminent. One patient felt much more secure when the recorder was on: it abated her fear of being seduced by the therapist and she had the security of being linked to the super-visor through the tape. Another way in which a comforting link can operate is in a clinic where therapists do not do their own assessments. Should it be the case that the supervisor did the entry assessment, and this fact is known to the patient, the result can be a reassuring sense of continuity and of not being lost in the organisation. Alternatively, that knowledge may accentuate feelings of having been abandoned and rejected by the assessor who, having heard the patient's story, did not

personally take him or her on for therapy. The patient's progress towards greater maturity may be evidenced in his or her attitude towards
being recorded. A self-preoccupied patient, who had refused taping
and who had difficulty in relating to others as whole persons, only
noticed after 3 years of therapy that her therapist had no index finger.
In a first show of concern for others, an important maturational stage,
she recognised that the lack of the finger would make writing up notes
difficult for him, and wished that she had agreed to being taped early in
therapy. Whatever the meaning, being taped is a significant event in
therapy and its meaning needs to be explored. Often when the therapeutic alliance is strong, taping will become a background issue, a
feature of the room rather than a feature of the therapy. However, the
position should be monitored by the therapist as the changing exploration of conflictual themes may propel the recorder centre-stage and
require its re-examination.

Confidentiality and Ethical Issues

Although in asking the patient for consent to tape the therapist may be
merely meeting the requirements of supervision, and have the admir-
able intent of advancing his understanding and performance, and
hence the effectiveness of his work with the patient, for the patient the
request may be abusive, or the experience of being taped too stressful
to be tolerated. The therapist needs to consider carefully the meaning
for the patient of being taped, and be aware of how easy it is to abuse
the power differential that always exists between therapist and patient.
The therapist's wish to tape must be tempered by the individual needs
of the patient.

Informed written consent is essential. In Nottingham, consent is
sought at the time of the assessment interview if this is to be taped, or
by the therapist near the beginning of the first session of therapy. The
therapist explains the purpose of taping and how the tapes will be
used. Our form of written consent is as follows:

Limited Consent Form
I consent to being audio/video-taped and I understand that the recording will
only be used for the purposes of supervision, teaching and evaluation within the
Psychotherapy Unit. I give my consent on the understanding that the recording
will be erased once the above purposes have been fulfilled or when my case
records are destroyed, whichever is the earlier, and that I may withdraw the
consent at any time and have the tape erased.
Name ....Signed .... Date ....
This agreement has been discussed with me by .... on ....

A copy of the consent is retained by the patient and a copy filed in the
case-notes. It is important that the consent is elective and can be with-

drawn at any time. If tapes are retained for teaching or research purposes for more than a year, consideration should be given to renewing the consent at appropriate intervals.

Additional consent should be sought if the tapes are to be used for purposes beyond that of limited consent. An example would be case presentations outwith the psychotherapy department at scientific meetings. The occasion should be described to the patient and an assurance given that a pledge of confidentiality will be given by the participants. In our *Extended Consent* form, an additional sentence reads: *I consent for the recordings to be used at professional meetings outside the Psychotherapy Unit where the participants have given a pledge of confidentiality.* When presenting the tape at the scientific meeting, the participants must be asked to give the pledge and to withdraw from the meeting if the patient is known to them in a personal capacity. The therapist or presenter should retain control of the tapes and should not allow them to be shown unless he is present. The only exception to this policy is when a teaching tape has been made and the patient(s) has given explicit consent for this exceptional use.

Special care should be taken to keep tapes secure, both physically and in terms of identification. It is not advisable to write the patient's name on the tape as this only advertises the identity of the recordee. Initials or a coded number should be used instead. Tapes should be wiped clean when no longer required.

Making Recordings

Recordings are at their most acceptable to the patient if they are routine and unobtrusive. These principles help the therapist contend with the process of being recorded. From the point of view of the supervisor, high-quality recordings are essential and video-tape is more interesting and informative than audio-tape. Poor-quality sound or vision quickly alienates.

For sound recordings, lapel microphones linked to the recorder by lead or radio wave provide the best quality sound. They are intrusive and have to be fitted and removed before and after each session. An omnidirectional or two-directional microphone placed on a table near the therapist and patient come next in order of unobtrusiveness. If a two-channel sound mixer is available, sound levels for each microphone can be adjusted to compensate for loud and quiet voices. A preferable solution is to use directional boom microphones, ideally with a zoom control so as to cut out extraneous sound, mounted on stands and placed on the other side of the room. Tapes should be longer than the anticipated duration of the sessions in order to avoid interrupting the flow of the session by having to turn the tape over; in individual psychotherapy, 60 minutes should be sufficient. A recorder with Dolby noise-reduction and bass and treble controls is advantageous.

The advent of inexpensive, easy to operate video-recorders which do not require high light levels means that this preferable medium is a viable choice for most psychotherapy departments. A recorder with a zoom lens and a zoom microphone can be mounted on a tripod across the room, giving either a lateral picture or a view of the patient over the therapist's shoulder. Video-8 tape is compact, gives high-quality recordings, and in extended play will record for 3 hours. To record group therapy, at least two static cameras are required, with the result being mixed on a split screen, each camera giving a view of half the group. A better system is to have a mobile camera operated by a technician who can follow the interaction and give close-ups, but this is obtrusive. Audio-tapes of group sessions are by and large incomprehensible.

Finding the correct position on the tape during supervision is difficult. For both audio- and video-tape, it is desirable to have equipment with real-time counters and a facility for memory marking the tape, either at the time or later.

After consent has been given, it is best to have the tape running before the session begins. Last-minute technical problems are avoided and the intrusive presence of the recorder is minimised. Some therapists time their 45-minute therapy sessions by using a 45-minute audio-tape. This has the undesirable effect of shattering whatever stage has been reached at the end of the session when the tape-recorder noisily switches itself off. On a countertransference level, the therapist may be avoiding dealing with the patient's hate over the session ending by displacing responsibility for ending from himself onto the machine. It is important to preserve the right of the patient to have the machine turned off at any moment that he does not want recorded.

Other Uses of Recordings

Having overcome the difficulties in making recordings, tapes may be used to enhance the effectiveness of therapy and for research and clinical audit. For example, a key element in the success of focal or brief psychotherapy is the identification of a dynamic focus of central importance to the patient, which is then worked with. In both Strupp's and Luborsky's model, the focus is derived from narrative statements made by the patient about the pattern of their relationships (Strupp and Binder, 1984; Luborsky and Crits-Christoph, 1990). In its pure form, Luborsky's core conflictual relationship themes are identified from content analysis of narrative segments from audio-tapes of sessions early and late in therapy. This labour-intensive procedure, involving as it does the services of independent identifiers of narrative segments and separate judges of the three elements in the theme – namely wish, expected response from others and consequent response to self – can only be sustained in a research programme. Nevertheless the procedure can be adapted to ordinary clinical practice. Narrative statements can be identified and their constituent elements teased out in supervision.

A more radical procedure in terms of altering the frame of therapy is the method of brief structured recall (Elliott and Shapiro, 1988) which is being used to good effect in research to elucidate what the patient judges to be the most significant event(s) in a session. The identified events are located on the audio-tape and the preceding and subsequent interactions and the event itself subjected to microanalysis of meaning and process by the patient and researcher or therapist. Undertaking this exercise from time to time is most instructive for the therapist; discrepancies in view are highlighted, and the therapist's awareness of the significance of his interaction and what is important to the patient is deepened. Certainly, undertaking this exercise predicates a collaborative style of working which may conflict with the style of less interactive forms of dynamic psychotherapy, but the price may be worth paying. It may be recalled that Alfred Adler used to meet with patient and therapist when therapy was stuck, for a three-way examination of what the problem was, without any apparent ill effect.

The methods detailed above may be used for clinical audit. They provide a quantifiable index of dynamically significant change.

Just as the one-way screen family therapy is now being used as an active element in therapy (Cade and Cornwell, 1985), so may tapes contribute to the therapeutic effect. Tapes can be lent to the patient for their private review after important sessions. Timing is of the essence, particularly if video-tape is borrowed, because the visual impact of that medium is great. A premature view may damage self-esteem by reinforcing negative perceptions of the self. It is more encouraging to view video-tape after several weeks or months have elapsed when, one predicts, change will be evident. An exception is in couple therapy where video feedback of problematic interactions can be very helpful. Occasionally, a patient will want to tape the sessions for himself!

Tapes, provided that the patient has given explicit consent, can form the basis of a teaching library. For example, how to conduct an assessment interview, begin a therapy session, and make an interpretation, can be illustrated.

Conclusion

Tapes have theoretical and practical disadvantages; however, they give direct access to the therapy session without the distortions of recollection. Perhaps their greatest value is in private review by the therapist. In supervision, they facilitate the close examination of process and technique. Discrepancies between the recollected account and the record are highlighted, not with the purpose of showing up the deficiencies of the therapist but as phenomena that have meaning and significance. How the therapist deals with transference and emotionally charged issues can be seen and discussed. Tapes are a useful, if not essential, aid in the supervision of dynamic psychotherapy.

The meaning of being taped needs to be carefully considered and monitored by the therapist. Taping should be used selectively and sensitively. Careful attention needs to be given to consent, confidentiality and the security of the tapes. These strictures and the importance of dynamic processes apply equally to behavioural and family therapy as to dynamic psychotherapy.

Acknowledgements

I would like to thank the participants in the Second Tavistock Symposium for the lively debates, and I thank Dr P. Slack for her comments on the manuscript.

References

BION, W. (1967). Notes on memory and desire. *Psychoanalytic Forum* 2, 272–280.

BROMBERG, P.M. (1984). The third ear. In: L. Caligor, P.M. Bromberg and J.D. Meitzer (Eds) *Clinical Perspectives on the Supervision of Psychoanalysis and Psychotherapy*. New York: Plenum Press.

CADE, B. and CORNWELL, M. (1985). New realities for old: some uses of teams and one-way screens in therapy. In: D. Campbell and R. Draper (Eds) *Applications of Systemic Family Therapy. The Milan Approach*. London: Grune & Stratton.

CALIGOR, L. (1984). Parallel and reciprocal processes in psychoanalytic supervision. In: L. Caligor, P.M. Bromberg and J.D. Meltzer (Eds) *Clinical Perspectives on the Supervision of Psychoanalysis and Psychotherapy*. New York: Plenum Press.

DOEHRMAN, M.J.G. (1976) Parallel processes in supervision and psychotherapy. *Bulletin of the Menninger Clinic* 40, 1–104.

ELLIOTT, R. and SHAPIRO, D.A. (1988). Brief structured recall: a more efficient method for studying significant therapy moments. *British Journal of Medical Psychology* 61, 141–153.

FLEMING, J. and BENEDEK, T. (1966). *Psychoanalytic Supervision: A Method of Clinical Teaching*. New York: International Universities Press.

FREUD, S. (1912). *Recommendations to Physicians Practicing Psychoanalysis*, standard edn, Vol. 12. London: Hogarth Press.

GUGGENBUHL-CRAIG, A. (1971). *Power in the Helping Professions*. Irving, TX: Spring Publications.

LUBORSKY, L. and CRITS-CHRISTOPH, P. (1990). *Understanding Transference. The CCRT Method*. New York: Basic Books.

REIK, T. (1949). *Listening with the Third Ear*. New York: Farrer, Straus.

RIOCH, M.J. (1980). The dilemmas of supervision in dynamic psychotherapy. In: A.K. Hess (Ed.) *Psychotherapy Supervision: Theory, Research and Practice*. New York: Wiley.

RIOCH, M.J., COULTER, W.R. and WEINBERGER, D.M. (1976). *Dialogues for Therapists*. San Francisco: Josey-Bass.

STRUPP, H.H. and BINDER, J.L. (1984). *A Guide to Time-Limited Dynamic Psycho-therapy*. New York: Basic Books.

WOLBERG, L.R. (1988). *The Technique of Psychotherapy*, 4th edn, Chapter 61. New York: Grune & Stratton.

Chapter 13
Issues in the Training of Group Therapists

Introduction

The book in which this first appeared documents the considerable variation that exists between different modalities of group approach; some are more cognitive, some more behavioural, some stress intrapsychic processes and some emphasise interpersonal transactions and the search for meaning. In some, the prime role of the leader is that of analyst or interpreter of the social matrix, in others, facilitator of interpersonal transactions, director or educator. Just as the emphasis will appeal differentially to members and will inform their choice of group should they be so fortunate as to have a variety to choose from, so will the different formats provide settings where the substantial variation between therapists can find fruitful expression. If the aim of therapy, as I believe, is to assist with the process of individuation and the development of the capacity to love and to work, then the therapist needs to know himself and recognise in what direction his talents lie.

Training should help the therapist make explicit his model of help-giving, examine how it may be integrated with the group situation, and identify natural preferences that may obstruct his therapeutic role (Lakin, Lieberman and Whitaker, 1969).

At this point, I must declare my bias towards interpersonal and analytic small groups. These modalities provide a rich conceptual framework for understanding the interpersonal and group processes that are present in all groups, and which may be harnessed in the therapeutic service of the group. I contend that whatever direction the natural talent of the trainee group therapist finally takes, his later performance will benefit from a close familiarity with these modalities early in training. They will provide a frame of reference against which special

From Aveline, M.O. (1988). Issues in the training of group therapists. In M.O. Aveline and W. Dryden (Eds), *Group Therapy in Britain*. Milton Keynes: Open University Press.

approaches may be deployed; the frame may or may not be explicitly referred to in practice, but is there to be drawn on in case of need. It follows that a suitable foundation experience would be as leader of a closed small-group meeting for 18 months; the same point is made by Yalom (1985). Moving from a specialised format to a general perspective is much more difficult once perceptual sets and practice habits have been established.

For the above reasons, the major focus of this chapter is on small-group psychotherapy. Most of the points made come from that field whose training literature, in contrast to others, is conspicuously systematic in its coverage. Although different approaches will need to teach the specifics of their way, the issues raised by the orthodox group therapy trainings have implications for the entire field.

This chapter first considers the qualities of the good leader, which are to be looked for in the trainee and brought out by the training; these are on two planes, one in personal characteristics and the other in the ability to conceptualise on several levels. Secondly, the typical problems of inexperienced leaders are described, because this is the point whence training begins. Thirdly, the elements that make up a balanced training are critically examined, together with some comments on the perspective of the leader. These sections are addressed to trainers as much as to trainees. Finally, advice is given on chosing a training.

The Good Leader

Personal characteristics

In general terms, the good leader will be characterised by an abiding interest in people, a fundamental conviction that people have it within them to change and to grow, and significantly, that group members can assist each other in this endeavour. In his interactions he should embody these attitudes; the good model he presents to the group is essential to the therapeutic process. He should enjoy being in the group, that is, once the severe anxiety that afflicts all group leaders early in their career has abated. He must have a highly ethical attitude.

As Grotjahn (1983) says, the ideal therapist must be reliable, as only then will he invite trust and confidence; he must trust and have confidence in himself and in others; he must be an expert in communication and a master of dynamic reasoning. In his interactions within the group, the leader needs to be spontaneous and responsive; being responsive also means being responsible. Though the leader will reflect upon the session afterwards, in the moment-to-moment exchange within the group he will need to respond honestly, openly and intuitively. Such spontaneity is bedded in trust and depends upon courage and the ability to withstand bad experiences without despair. A firm identity, the capacity to identify with others, the ability to laugh at oneself and acknowledge mistakes, and a willingness to be a bystander in the interactive focus complete this portrait. The picture is far distant from the harmful profile identified by Lieberman, Yalom and Miles (1973) in their meticulous study of psychological casualties among members of encounter groups led by experienced leaders. Leaders who were intrusive and aggressive and who demanded rapid self-disclosure, emotional expression and attitude change, when combined with members who were particularly vulnerable or who had unrealistic expectations, accounted for all but one of the casualties, who totalled 9 per cent of the sample of 219 subjects. The leader who is aloof and distant also contributes to negative effects (Dies and Teleska, 1985).

The complexity of a therapy group far exceeds that of individual therapy. Whereas in the latter the therapist has to strive to comprehend the conscious and unconscious selves of one person, in the group the database is multiplied eightfold or more. Furthermore, the group as a whole has a reality whose form illuminates individual and shared personal difficulties, and which, in most approaches, needs to be addressed if the full potential of the group for therapeutic change is to be realised. In contrast to individual therapy, the leader achieves the therapeutic effect in work with and through group members, rather than directly out of the single relationship between the therapist and patient or help-seeker. For some, these elements constitute the attraction of group work; for others, the complexity and the seemingly inevitable chaos is aversive.

Whilst training may improve the competence of the leader by increasing knowledge, inculcating skills and reducing defensive personal strategies which may inhibit the good development of the group, there is no evidence that training itself can remedy a basic lack of aptitude for group work. For those with aptitude, much hard work needs to be done before the craft of group leadership is learnt, and the reward of fully using this powerful instrument for improving interpersonal relationships is gained.

An individual and a collective perspective

In judging whether or not and how to intervene, the leader of a small therapy group needs to examine what is happening in the group from several perspectives. These are assessed against the context of (1) the developmental stage and (2) the history of the group. Thus the priorities of the leader will vary with the stage of the group; in the beginning, building a secure, cohesive base and establishing facilitative ground-rules will be the dominant task; later, once a working group is formed, fine tuning and a gentle insistence that termination issues be faced may be the chief activity. Similarly, the history and composition of the group will weight the leader's decisions – a group that scapegoats and punishes will require different corrective action from one that cannot tolerate sadness. Also, possible interventions are subject to two overriding principles: (1) what is the most emotionally charged issue, and (2) what intervention in the best judgement of the leader would be most likely to facilitate the fruitful development of the group? Generally, it may be said that the good functioning of the group as a whole takes precedence over individual concerns.

To illustrate the complexity of the dual perspective ideally required of the leader, a schema of the decision-making process is presented.

1. The leader takes an individual and a collective perspective.
2. The leader attends to process as well as content, both in the individuals and in the group.
3. *Content* delineates surface concerns which have a certain importance. They may contain the individual's and the group's understanding of what the difficulties are, what they signify and how they have come about.
4. *Process* reveals the nature of the underlying fears that unconsciously move the group as a whole, or mobilise defensive strategies in the individual or prompt him or her to tell a story which indirectly conveys an experienced but unacceptable feeling.
5. Thus, the leader needs to remember:
   (a) the history of the group, its drama, personalities and stage;
   (b) the histories of the members, their particular sensitivities and concerns;
   (c) the sequence of interactions, feelings and focus within members and within the group from one session to the next, and from moment to moment within the session.
6. The leader attends to the content and the process of the session, facilitating its expression, its exploration, and looking for shared central themes.
7. Furthermore, the leader derives an understanding of what are the important, perhaps unrecognised, issues in the group, by being aware of his inner feelings, by recognising the role-relationships that the group and members encourage him into, and by noticing the emotionally charged issues that the group and the individual avoid.
8. The leader considers the relationship of the group as a social system to the larger social and institutional systems of which it is a part, and between which there is a two-way exchange (Kernberg, 1975). The leader considers the group in its context.
9. From the above the leader decides to intervene individually or collectively, or to wait for the situation to clarify itself, or,

frequently, to wait for the group to act, bearing in mind the developmental stage of the group, its strengths and the personalies of its members.

It is recognised that this schema will be modified by the imperatives of different forms of group therapy.

Inexperienced Leaders and Their Problems

The inexperienced leader often has difficulty in making sense of what is happening in the group. In part, this is a function of the immense size of the phenomenal field in group therapy, but also he is subject to strong emotional pressures. The group may be hostile or resistant; it may doubt his competence. The relationship with the co-leader or leaders may be tenuous or frankly rivalrous. Colleagues may doubt the validity of what is being done and professional standing may be in jeopardy. Supervision itself may be a further source of performance anxiety. Hopefully the leader will be sustained by positive, expert supervision, having seen more experienced therapists at work and achieving good results, or the internalised memory of a good personal group experience, but sometimes this will not be the case.

The views of 100 experienced supervisors on the difficulties experienced by inexperienced group therapists were elicited by Dies (1980a). The two most frequent problems were insensitivity to group process and inappropriately attempting to do individual therapy in a group setting; this may be a function of greater familiarity with individual therapy among leaders before commencing group training. Role problems, in particular of being overactive – in other words, overstructuring as a way of containing the therapist's anxiety – or being excessively concerned with projecting a competent or powerful image, and countertransference fears of scapegoating or being unable to confront intense group issues, followed in rank order. Technical errors, such as in the form or timing of interpretations and inaccurate preparation for the role, were less frequently mentioned. Similar findings have been previously reported. As well as emphasising the burdensome sense of responsibility that the leader has for the group. Brody (1966) pointed to conflicts over the degree of therapist transparency. The six fearful fantasies identified by Williams (1966) were (1) encountering unmanageable resistance, (2) losing control of the group, (3) excessive hostility breaking out, (4) acting out by members, (5) overwhelming dependency demands on the leader and (6) the group disintegrating. Hunter and Stern (1968) focused on problems within the supervision group; these included fear of exposure and criticism by peers and the supervisor, threats to self-esteem and sibling rivalry.

As well as the acquisition of complex cognitive and technical skills, group training must take full account of the powerful emotional reactions of leaders to their role. The term 'leaders' is deliberately used without the qualifier of 'inexperienced', as experience does not, and probably should not, armour the leader against the tension of the moment. Too much tension narrows the therapeutic vision of the leader, too little robs him of the spur to creativity.

Elements in a Balanced Training

Supervised experience of leading groups, knowledge of theory and some form of personal experience in groups are the three elements that form the bedrock of training in group therapy (Larkin et al., 1969; Dies, 1980a,b). Observing experienced leaders at work is generally considered valuable. However, the utility of solo versus co-leadership, of being the junior leader, of being for training purposes a member of a patient group rather than a professional group, and the necessity of prior training in individual therapy are hotly debated issues. This section critically examines the elements that enter into a balanced training.

Supervised practice

The small group has a character of its own, similar to, but in important ways different from, a large group or a community meeting; the differences are much accentuated by the purpose and theoretical orientation of the leader. It is self-evident that the trainee must gain experience in the modality of the group in which he is seeking to become proficient. However, as has been stated, there is much to be said for the foundation experience as leader of a small closed group with a duration of 12–18 months; group processes are easier to perceive and their recurrent nature allows interventions to be practised and evaluated, the trainee can live through the natural history of a group from its hesitant beginnings at the selection stage to the dispersal of the members at the end, and with good supervision and member selection the chance of an encouraging initiation to group work is enhanced. I regret that in my experience all too many potential leaders begin and quickly end their careers by attempting to lead unstructured, unsupervised large groups, often on in-patient or day-patient psychiatric units which have made a token investment in group therapy.

It is preferable to gain experience of solo and co-leadership, as each form has advantages and disadvantages. Trainees of the Institute of Group Analysis in London are required to be solo leaders of their training group. Responsibility for what happens within the meeting is clearly theirs and must serve as a powerful concentrator of the mind; evaluation of that trainee's performance is made easier. On the other hand, the processes of the group are so complex and at times the pressures so great – when, for example, the group unites against the leader – that a co-leader is a welcome additional observer and ally. Furthermore, the presence of a co-leader facilitates the good practice of reflecting on the recent history of the group before the session, and reviewing the events of the meeting immediately afterwards. At times one co-leader will, by intention or experience, be junior to the other; this fact contributes its own oedipal dynamic to the group and may need to be focused on by the supervisor. Occasionally, a trainee may be placed in the room as a silent observer; this role is tenable for a brief period prior to assuming the responsibilities of leadership, but otherwise soon becomes boring.

Proper record keeping is essential. This may take the form of a chronogram (Cox, 1973): the time sequence of the meeting is represented by quadrants of a circle, key interactions are noted in the appropriate segment and arrows used to link themes and active members. The author favours a written naturalistic narrative of the session which documents the form and sequence of the interactions, the feelings that were present and the interventions of the leader; countertransference feelings and hypotheses about the group process may be included (Bloch et al., 1975). Alternatively, a structured report identifying key themes, group and individual interactions and leadership issues may be compiled (see Chapter 14). Circulating the written reports to group members may form part of the therapy (Yalom, Brown and Bloch, 1975).

For the purposes of supervision, written reports may be supplemented by audio or video recording of the group meetings. The technical quality of the recordings in both modalities needs to be very high if they are to be usable. For audio recordings, an overhead microphone or preferably several centrally placed directional microphones, whose inputs can be individually adjusted for the quiet or noisy group member, are necessary. A technician-controlled two-camera system is ideal for video recordings; whole-group shots should be used sparingly because rarely do they provide sufficient detail to hold the viewer's attention; medium shots and zoomed close-ups are much better. Recordings provide information on the non-verbal communications of members and leaders alike, whose comprehension is so important in the practice of group therapy.

The supervisor should be involved from the outset. Improved outcome is the reward of careful preparation. The supervisor should clarify the purpose and form of the proposed group and anticipate with the leaders the problems they are likely to encounter; role-play may be a useful way of working through the latter (see below). Selection and preparation of members is equally important – the former to maintain the principle of heterogeneity of personal style and homogeneity of severity of problem, and the latter to reduce the incidence of drop-out in the early phase of the group.

The supervisor will help the leaders acquire the individual and collective perspective previously outlined in this chapter. Two, or even three, pairs of co-leaders sharing a supervisory 1½ hours provide peer support, a further opportunity for multiple perspectives on the same event and the chance to see how similar therapeutic dilemmas are handled differently.

To help the supervisor register the cast of characters and understand the unique flavour of that group, a wise move is to observe the first one or two sessions and, if so desired, to repeat this periodically. Yalom's (1985) counsel of perfection is to observe the last 30 minutes of each session and then hold the supervisory meeting immediately afterwards.

Theory and the question of prior training in individual therapy

The theory component of a training should be comprehensive in scope, coherent in logic and critical of the tenets which underlie or are assumed to underlie the particulars of that approach. The last may be too much to ask of committed trainers in a training scheme but it is still the ideal. Often trainings are too narrow in their conceptual base and ignore the overlapping and complementary perspectives of knowledge held by other schools. Trainers tend to overvalue the validity of their approach. It is worth bearing in mind that the best estimate of the contribution made by technique to outcome across psychotherapies is only 15 per cent (Lambert, 1985). Until it can be demonstrated that certain techniques contribute a much higher percentage to the variance, the sage therapist will resist the siren call of a narrow but comfortingly secure theoretical base, and instead listen to many songs before, in a critical spirit, composing a melody that tells the truth as it is then known.

It has been suggested that only some therapists will be suited to group work. Dies, in several surveys of the literature (Dies, 1980a; Dies and Teleska, 1985), makes the point that many inexperienced group therapists do not appreciate the nature of the therapeutic factors that uniquely operate in groups (e.g. altruism, self-disclosure to peers and feedback), and hence do not make use of them. In part, this may be a function of prior orientation to and training in individual therapy. In the past, group training programmes have frequently emerged from institutes primarily concerned with individual therapy (Laking et al., 1969). Psychoanalysis has been the starting point for many group therapists; it has drawn attention to unconscious processes that contribute to the formation of the social matrix of the group, and highlighted the transferential relationship between the leader or conductor, in the terminology of the British Group-Analytic Society, and the members. For Pines (1979), analysis is a primary discipline in training. Similarly, Grotjahn (1983) speaks of the group psychotherapist coming from an analytic background, but points especially to how in the maturation of that therapist a personal group analysis will attend to the unanalysed family romance. In its training guidelines, the American Group Psychotherapy Association recommends ten times as many hours' supervised practice in individual therapy as in group therapy (1200–120 hours), whilst the Institute of Group Analysis in Britain, though being interested in a candidate's previous analysis or experience as a therapist, only requires group experience. Evaluative research should be carried out to elucidate the value in group therapy training of prior or concurrent training in individual therapy.

Personal experience as a group member

In learning to be a group leader, the personal experience of being a group member completes the training triad of supervised practice and theoretical learning. All three are essential and inseparable. The lived experience of being a member of a group not only makes sense of the theory but has the greatest chance of being integrated into the developing professional identity of the leader if it parallels in time the presentation of a comprehensive conceptual framework (Dies, 1980b). The intention of the experience is to deepen awareness of the group process, enhance self-knowledge and foster sensitivity to the needs and feelings of others (see Chapter 9); it provides an opportunity to experience a climate of openness and enquiry, and a chance to increase the ability of the participants to be innovative (Berger, 1970). Thus it is not surprising that all major training programmes in group therapy require a personal group experience.

The Institute of Group Analysis requires candidates for the qualifying course, its most advanced training which leads to full membership of the Group-Analytic Society, to undergo a personal group analysis in a twice-weekly group throughout the 3 years or more of training; the group is a patient-group, with trainee members being most definitely in the minority. The duration of the group analysis is about right for a specialist professional qualification, but the requirement for membership of a patient-group requires comment. In its favour is the fact that the patient role is experienced in its entirely; on practical grounds, it is, perhaps, easier to organise entry to a therapy group meeting for 3 years than to have available a sufficient number of trainee groups; and the anonymity of such a group may facilitate the exploration of personal issues without loss of face – certainly, sibling rivalry and concern about being judged by fellow professionals is reduced (Bathegay, 1983). However, the presence of a trainee, albeit as a full member, introduces a powerful dynamic whose resolution may be long drawn-out; spy, *agent provocateur* and leader's assistant are some of the roles that may be ascribed or assumed. Furthermore, the health care professional has some special preoccupations which need attending to during training.

In an analysis of personal themes raised by health care professionals in 21 12-week closed training groups that formed part of an introductory course for group leaders, found that a number of themes recurred (see Chapter 9). Many members took the opportunity to reveal personal tragedies that they felt could not be expressed at work for fear of being thought weak. They feared damaging their careers by self-disclosure. In their work-role as helper, they often felt unappreciated and helpless; in the group, they were able to express their experience that giving care and not receiving it was ultimately burdensome (McCarley, 1975). Just as in any therapy group, but given special poignancy by the fact that the majority of members worked in mental health and hence might be expected to be more insightful, the exploration of these personal and professional issues was obstructed by the initial tendency of members to see each other in stereotype and not as people. Despite the brief life of the group, many members entered into intimate dialogue with colleagues, sometimes for the first time; others were supported through personal crises or helped to make career decisions.

Provided that the group is well composed in terms of heterogeneity of coping style and homogeneity of severity of interpersonal difficulty, membership of a patient-group affords the most realistic setting for personal learning, and is to be preferred for advanced levels of professional training. However, there should also be an opportunity to explore the issues of the professional role in a group of mental health care colleagues.

In the training of group therapists, there is room for exposure to a variety of approaches and durations. An introductory 3-month or 1-year personal group experience is sufficient to acquaint a trainee with the nature of the modality and, more importantly, to determine if this is the direction in which the therapist's talents lie. Intensive 1-day or residential workshops are useful (for an example, see Lerner, Horwitz and Bernstein, 1978), but it is only through repeated experience over a longer period that the natural rhythm of hard-won personal change can be learnt.

The leader of the training group is in a position of influence and responsibility. The style of the leader is likely to be internalised – at least for a while – and the sensitivity and professionalism with which personal issues and intragroup conflicts are handled will enhance or detract from the trainee's liking for the approach. The leader needs to be chosen with care. Yalom (1985) suggests that the determining factors are talent, experience and, for the first training group, a non-specialised format. In the interests of confidentiality and to underline the fact that the organisers of the training programme will not have access to any evaluation made by the leader, the leader should be clearly seen to be independent of the training organisation (Berman, 1975; Shapiro, 1978; Dies, 1980a; Yalom, 1985).

Role-play and observing experienced therapists at work

In a promising development, British group analysts have formulated a series of problematic group scenarios as part of an investigation into how different leaders may conceptualise and intervene in the group (Garland et al., 1984). The discussion of these scenarios with trainees is a useful teaching aid. Issues may be explored without putting group members at risk. The exercise can be extended by role-playing the issue and then soliciting feedback from participants and observers; the techniques of psychodrama, namely role rehearsal and reversal, auxiliary ego and de-roling, can be used advantageously to elucidate the minutiae of the interaction. Role-play is a flexible technique which can be adjusted to the needs of inexperienced and advanced trainees (Lakin et al., 1969). Further details of structured exercises may be found in MacLennan (1971), Cohen and Smith (1976) and Roman and Porter (1978).

The essence of learning is doing and reflecting on what was done, but seeing can accelerate the process. Observing experienced group leaders at work has relatively low priority in group training, perhaps because of the passive status of the observer (Dies, 1980b). However, as Shapiro (1978) comments, observing a professional leader presents a golden opportunity to get a realistic picture of the true nature of group leadership; successes and failures can be seen, the results of specific interventions in specific situations examined and the whole put in the context of the trainee's developing skills as a leader. Yalom (1985) strongly advocates observation of a group for a minimum of 4 months, preferably from behind a one-way screen, the sessions being followed by 30–45 minutes of discussion between the leader(s) and the observers. This exacting task benefits both parties. If resources allow, a trainer can sit with the observers during the sessions and draw attention to the multiple elements entering into each interaction. As with individual supervision, the discussion period can degenerate into the post hoc cleverness of 'why didn't you do this or that?' instead of examining the issues and leadership dilemmas. For this reason, some trainers prefer to have the trainees each write an account of the session which brings out the interpersonal processes that they observed and have this as the basis of the discussion later in the week. Dies (1980b) lists ten scales that can be completed by observers, five of which focus on leadership and five on group process; these scales help structure the trainees' attention. The discussion period offers an opportunity to learn how to give clear feedback in a sensitive, supportive manner, a skill whose necessity will be sharply underlined if leaders and students reverse their roles in another training exercise later in the programme.

Observing a group is always a privilege. Few if any group members welcome being observed and some feel persecuted by it. The reactions of members form another focus for exploration, but it must not be forgotten that they are being asked to accept an intrusion and that the final decision has to be theirs. Permission must be sought to have observers, and when someone is behind the one-way screen, their presence must be declared; some groups prefer to meet briefly with any new observer so that their presence is less anonymous. The situation needs to be handled with sensitivity and tact; observers arriving late and the sound of laughter are simple examples of what should not happen. Borrowing a practice from therapeutic communities, the fish bowl, the group can be offered the opportunity to change rooms and observe the post-group discussion. If this is done, it is important that all members attend; in my experience, the interest of members in this extra dimension is short-lived. Once the persecutory fantasies have been dispelled and voyeuristic interest satisfied, members prefer to use their time in other ways. The fish bowl procedure demystifies group therapy and would easily integrate with most of the approaches described in this book; it might, however, be dissonant with group analysis with its greater emphasis on transference.

Evaluation

Training without evaluation is a lost opportunity for learning and an abnegation of responsibility by the trainers. At an introductory level, a certificate of attendance may be all that is looked for. At an advanced level, completion of the training should be a statement of quality and should be marked by a normative evaluation; it must be possible for trainees to fail or be deferred. At all levels, there is room for repeated formative evaluations which help the trainee make fuller use of the subsequent training. In the group course organised by the author, a written, tentative evaluation of their strengths and weaknesses as potential group leaders is sent by the leader to each member of the training group at its mid-point; the comments may be worked on in subsequent sessions (see Chapter 14).

The entry and evaluation procedures at the Institute of Group Analysis for the qualifying course is an excellent example of a carefully applied professional system, and so is described in detail. The involvement of many members of the Institute in the procedures introduces a system of checks and balances. Candidates first meet with a consultant for a personal assessment and then with the Board of Assessors, whose report is considered by the Admission Sub-Committee before a final decision on entry is made by the Training Committee. Any deficiencies in experience are identified and candidates may be advised, for example, to seek a period of individual therapy before entering training, or to gain experience with major psychiatric illness if coming from a lay background. Admission to seminars comes after about 1 year's membership of a therapy group and a satisfactory report from the group analyst. This report, together with seminar leaders' reports, forms the key elements in the decision of the Training Committee to allow the student to conduct a weekly group under supervision. Any element in the training may be extended; supervisors', seminar leaders' and group analyst's reports contribute to the assessment that training is complete. The metaphor of the training is that the student is on a personal and professional journey, and that by sharing the evaluations with the student at each stage, the journey can be facilitated.

In common with other psychotherapy trainings, objective criteria of competence, and in particular of the therapeutic effectiveness, are lacking. At the end of the day, a global gut feeling that the trainee is an ethical, competent therapist to whom one might safely entrust one's nearest and dearest is, I suspect, the deciding factor in the evaluator's mind. There is much to be said for retaining this as the fundamental construct in designing courses and evaluating outcomes.

Research

It is a counsel of perfection to expect trainees to be personally involved in conducting research. However, as has been stated, it is important that the trainee maintains a critical (but not cynical) attitude to what is being taught. Organisers of training programmes should ensure that their students are acquainted with the findings from research, and help them consider what implications they may have for practice. Certainly the trainee should be familiar with research methodology and may find it helpful in their learning about therapeutic factors, group development and group processes, to apply the research instruments of the major studies to their own group or observed group.

The perspective of the supervisor and his training

The supervisor, though only participating in the groups at second hand, has the great advantage of hindsight and a certain psychological distance from the action. These two elements, together with the wisdom of clinical experience and depth of theoretical knowledge, are brought to bear on the responsible task of facilitating learning. As has been advocated, the supervisor should be closely involved from the outset. Just as the leader of a group fosters helpful group norms and draws attention to important but neglected aspects of the group exchange, so does the supervisor attend to aspects that are not fully in view by the trainee. Bascue (1978) suggests eight therapeutic dimensions that need to be considered: past and present, external and internal, cognitive and affective, verbal and behavioural, individual and group, leader and member activity, manifest and latent meaning, problem solving and personality change. I stress the importance of the individual, collective and contextual perspectives.

Training for supervision is a neglected issue. To be made a supervisor on an established course is an honour, but rarely is preparation given for this role or support continued as the supervisor hones his skills. Several precautionary steps can be taken. Two supervisors leading a supervisory seminar may learn from each other as well as offering different perspectives; a junior supervisor may serve an apprenticeship period with a more experienced one. Written yearly evaluations by the supervisee of the supervisor and vice versa ensures that an appraisal is made of the work that has been done. Problems in supervision should be discussed at regular meetings of supervisors. Finally, the exacting challenge of leading a training group of experienced therapists is an excellent postgraduate training (Grotjahn, 1983).

Guidelines in Selecting a Training

At an advanced level, the leader will know what kind of group work he is most suited to and will seek training in that, but the beginner has a greater need for variety. The foregoing sections offer a guide to what a trainee might look for in a training. The principal points are now reiterated. Trainings which offer the opportunity to experience and evaluate critically their approach are to be preferred. The training should provide extensive practice as a leader with more than one supervisor. Theory should be comprehensively taught and high ethical and normative standards adhered to. A personal group experience should be offered, as should the opportunity to observe and discuss the work of experienced leaders. Commitment to a training should only follow the affirmative answering of the private question: 'Will this training help me to know more clearly what my talents are as a therapist and develop them?'

References

BASCUE, I.O. (1978). A conceptual model for training group therapists. *International Journal of Group Psychotherapy* **28**, 445–452.

BATHEGAY, R. (1983). The value of analytic self-experiencing in the training of psychotherapists. *International Journal of Group Psychotherapy* **33**, 199–213.

BERGER, M.M. (1970). Experiential and didactic aspects of training in therapeutic group approaches. *American Journal of Psychiatry* **126**, 840–845.

BERMAN, A.L. (1975). Group psychotherapy training. *Small Group Behavior* **6**, 325–344.

BLOCH, S., BROWN, S., DAVIS, K. and DISHOTSKY, N. (1975). The use of a written summary in group psychotherapy supervision. *American Journal of Psychiatry* **132**, 1055–1057.

BRODY, L.S. (1966). Harrassed! A dialogue. *International Journal of Group Psychotherapy* **16**, 463–500.

COHEN, A.M. and SMITH, R.D. (1976). *The Critical Incident in Growth Groups: A Manual for Group Leaders*. LaJolla. California: University Associates.

COX, M. (1973). The group therapy interaction chronogram. *British Journal of Social Work* **3**, 243–256.

DIES, R.R. (1980a). Group psychotherapy: training and supervision. In: A.K. Hess (Ed.) *Psychotherapy Supervision: Theory, Research and Practice,* pp. 337–366. New York: Wiley.

DIES, R.R. (1980b). Current practice in the training of group psychotherapists. *International Journal of Group Psychotherapy* **30**, 169–185.

DIES, R.R. and TELESKA, P.A. (1985). Negative outcome in group psychotherapy. In D.T. Mays and C.M. Franks (Eds) *Negative Outcomes in Psychotherapy and What to Do About It,* pp. 118–141. New York: Springer.

GARLAND, C., KENNARD, O., ROBERTS, J.P., WINTER, D.A., CAINE, T.M., DICK, B. and STEVNESON, F.B. (1984). What is a group analyst? A preliminary investigation of conductor's interview. *Group Analysis* **17**, 137–145.

GROTJAHN, M. (1983). The qualities of the group therapist. In: H.I. Kaplan and B.J. Sadock (Eds) *Comprehensive Group Psychotherapy,* 2nd edn., pp. 249–301. Baltimore: Williams & Wilkins.

HUNTER, G.F. and STERN, H. (1968). The training of mental health workers. *International Journal of Group Psychotherapy* **28**, 104–109.

KERNBERG, O.F. (1975). A systems approach to priority setting of interventions in groups. *International Journal of Group Psychotherapy* **25**, 251–275.

LAKIN, M., LIEBERMAN, M. and WHITAKER, D. (1969). Issues in the training of group psychotherapists. *International Journal of Group Psychotherapy* **19**, 307–325.

LAMBERT, M.J. (1985). Implications of psychotherapy outcome research for eclectic psychotherapy. In: T.C. Norcross (Ed) *Handbook of Eclectic Psychotherapy,* pp. 436–462. New York: Brunner/Mazel.

LERNER, H.E., HORWITZ, L. and BURSTEIN, E.D. (1978). Teaching psychoanalytic group psychotherapy: a combined experiential didactic workshop. *International Journal of Group Psychotherapy* **28**, 453–466.

LIEBERMAN, M.A., YALOM, I.D. and MILES, M.B. (1973). *Encounter Groups: First Facts.* New York: Basic Books.

McCARLEY, T. (1975). The psychotherapist's search for self-renewal. *American Journal of Psychiatry* **132**, 221–224.

MacLENNAN, B.W. (1971). Simulated situations in group psychotherapy training. *International Journal of Group Psychotherapy* **21**, 330–332.

PINES, M. (1979). Group psychotherapy: frame of reference for training. *Group Analysis* **12**, 210–218.

ROMAN, M. and PORTER, K. (1978). Combining experiential and didactic aspects in a new group therapy training approach. *International Journal of Group Psychotherapy* **28**, 371–387.

SHAPIRO, J.E. (1978). *Methods of Group Psychotherapy and Encounter*. Itasca, IL: Peacock.

WILLIAMS, M. (1966). Limitations, fantasies and security operations of beginning group psychotherapists. *International Journal of Group Psychotherapy* **16**, 150–162.

YALOM, I.D. (1985). *The Theory and Practice of Group Psychotherapy*, 3rd edn. New York: Basic Books.

YALOM, I.D., BROWN, S. and BLOCH, S. (1975). The written summary as a group psychotherapy technique. *Archives of General Psychiatry* **32**, 605–613.

Chapter 14
The Use of Written Reports in a Brief Group Psychotherapy Training

Introduction

The use of a written summary mailed to members after each therapy session has been recommended by Yalom, Brown and Bloch (1975) as a group psychotherapy technique, and as an aid to supervision (Bloch et al., 1975).

In 1976 the author devised an annual introductory, multidisciplinary course which provides practical, systematic training for inexperienced group leaders in 12 weekly sessions. Ten courses have been held; 210 health care workers, mainly employed in the National Health Service, have taken the training. The course includes a closed training group experience with ten members in each group; the personal themes from these groups are described elsewhere (see Chapter 9). Written reports of the content of the group meetings have been an innovative, integral and valuable part of the learning process.

Written Reports

In this application, two approaches have been used; their evaluation has been by post-course questionnaire.

Courses 1–7

To link theory and practice, the leader of each T-group circulated to members after each meeting a detailed typewritten report, 1000–2000 words in length. The content of the report interwove three elements: (1) a naturalistic narrative; (2) the leader's view of the dynamics of both the group and individual members; and (3) an explanation of why the

From M.O. Aveline (1986) The use of written reports in a brief group psychotherapy training. *International Journal of Group Psychotherapy* 36, 477–482.

leader chose to intervene or not to intervene. In style the reports have emulated Yalom, Brown and Bloch's (1975) 'intimate picture of the therapist's unspoken observations, hunches, foibles, puzzlement and, at times, discouragement in therapy' (p. 605).

The members of these groups were preparing to be group leaders. They needed both to experience and to analyse what was happening. For the leader to step out of role during the session and become a teacher of leadership skills would have fragmented the experience. The reports separated the experience in the 'now' from the thinking about it in the 'then'. They took members behind the scenes and acquainted them with the dilemmas that the leader faced. Seeing what the leader felt and thought encouraged them to consider how they might act when leading a similar meeting. In our experience, revealing the mechanics of the group has not hindered the development of mature, cohesive working groups.

Receiving group reports has been universally welcomed. One member commented, 'I read them like a weekly instalment of my favourite childhood comic. I use them for reflection on issues and to measure my own perceptions with those in the reports. I use them for reassurance and for making sense of complex sessions'. Characteristically, the reports are read avidly in the early sessions, particularly for references to self. Later on, perhaps as members feel more confident in the acceptance they have gained within the group, the reports become less important, though they still remain a useful aide memoire. Members have found it particularly illuminating when the report has corrected perceptions of them either having said too much or too little about themselves or some issue during the meeting; the report has brought an external perspective which is hard for the protagonist to have for himself. However, there is a danger that by writing down exchanges, interactions and asides, a more conspicuous form is given to something that the member may have wanted to be half-heard. For a time, people may need to preserve the illusion that their secrets are secret (Meares, 1976).

Naturally, how members react to the report may be read on many levels, from the factual to the dynamic. Resistance and, in particular, hostility may first surface in dismissive and argumentative comments about the contents of the report, and was well put by one woman who said that she had used her report to write her shopping list on, and by another that she had wallpapered her room with them.

For a 1½-hour group, a further 1½ hours are required to prepare a report of this length; the time-commitment disadvantage is compounded by that of selectivity. It is impossible to remember all the events and nuances of a session, and the leader will have his own personal bias, overattending to certain events and avoiding others. Despite this, members have been generally complimentary about the accuracy of the reports and have at times fantasised a secret tape-recording of the meetings.

Through the group report, the leader may convey his affirmative concern, which is supportive. Alternatively the overt reinforcement of group norms and the selection of certain material over and against other material not only reveals the leader's intent, but can be experienced as coercive. It is easy to be overdefinitive and the format does not allow misunderstandings to be resolved as they happen. The leader may evade necessary tension and conflict by deferring to the report what should have been said in the session. Furthermore, negative feelings toward the group are hard to hide in the report.

Courses 8–10

For the above reasons, a four-question structured report by the leader, emphasising leadership skills, was introduced and circulated as before:

1. What themes were present in this session?
2. How were these themes tackled in the group?
3. How were these themes tackled by the leader?
4. How were members involved in the session?

Before the leader's report arrives, members complete their own report under the following headings:

1. What themes were present in the session and how were they tackled by the group?
2. What, in your view, was the most significant event, interaction or sequence in this session? Who was this most significant for?
3. Who, including yourself, was most involved in this session?
4. Who, including yourself, was least involved in this session?
5. What event was most *personally important* to you during this session? This might be something that involved you directly or something that happened between other members, but which made you think about yourself.
6. What in this session was particularly difficult for the leader as leader?

Question 5 is adapted from the Group Climate Questionnaire (Mackenzie, 1981).

After sessions 3 and 9, a copy of each member's report is sent to the other members of the training group.

This procedure retains the advantages of the original report, but the trainees are now much more actively involved in observing and analysing key events and problems, activities which are of great relevance to their future role as group leaders. Members may privately compare their perspective and the leader's perspective; these reports do not require further self-disclosure. By exchanging reports on two occasions, the individual is made vividly aware of how the same event is seen and felt differently by others. Convergence and perception tend to characterise the second sharing.

The new procedures have been well received. Neither leader nor members find the task of writing the reports too onerous. For the leader, the temptation remains to defer to the report what should have been said in the session, but the briefer format is a deterrent. Members value the opportunity to compare perspectives and to consider the problems of leadership as a separate exercise from being a group member.

Evaluation of the Potential of Members as Group Leaders

Training courses rarely evaluate the performance of the participants (Dies, 1980). In the last three courses, this important but difficult task has been attempted by the leader sending each member after session 6 a confidential, tentative evaluation of their potential as group leaders. Most members choose to discuss their evaluation in the group.

Receiving these evaluations is stressful. Trainees have reported delaying reading them for days, or even getting someone else to read them first. In reality, the evaluations are not persecutory, as the intention is to make enabling and occasionally challenging comments. Having the evaluation in written form ensures that the intended message can be received after the initial period of shock or relief has passed. Coming at the mid-point of the course, there is time to work on the interpersonal issues that have been raised. Often the evaluations have prompted more self-disclosure and greater cohesion. Our impression is that the reports and the evaluations strengthen the work of the group. This is in line with the positive value of feedback in a controlled study of brief therapy with married couples (Soeken et al., 1981).

Conclusion

Written reports and personal evaluations are useful adjuncts in teaching health care professionals to be group leaders. They complete the triangle of theory and personal experience by illuminating the doubts, uncertainties, dilemmas and gambles that the leader has to take. Having members complete their own reports promotes active learning and encourages them to anticipate problems that they will encounter as leaders.

References

BLOCH, S., BROWN, S., DAVIS, K. and DISHOTSKY, N. (1975). The use of a written summary in group psychotherapy supervision. *American Journal of Psychiatry* **132**, 1055–1057.

DIES, R.R. (1980). Current practice in the training of group psychotherapists. *International Journal of Group Psychotherapy* **30**, 169–185.

MACKENZIE, K.R. (1981). Measurement of group climate. *International Journal of Group Psychotherapy* **31**, 287–295.

MEARES, R. (1976). The secret. *Psychiatry* **39**, 258–265.

SOEKEN, D.R., MANDERSCHELD, R.W., FLATTER, C.H. and SILBERGELD, S. (1981). A controlled study of quantitative feedback in married couples brief group psychotherapy. *Psychotherapy, Theory, Research and Practice* **18**, 201–216.

YALOM, I., BROWN, S. and BLOCH, S. (1975). The written summary as a group psychotherapy technique. *Archives of General Psychiatry* **32**, 605–613.

Chapter 15
Developing a New NHS Psychotherapy Service and Training Scheme in the Provinces

Introduction

The early 1970s saw the beginning of a major investment by the National Health Service in specialist psychotherapy which continues to this day. The expansion was marked by a document from the Royal College of Psychiatrists (1975) which recommended staffing norms for psychotherapy services (now nationally half achieved) and the formal recognition of the medical specialty by the DHSS in 1978. Much of the expansion has taken place in the Provinces; its local form has been powerfully influenced by the conceptual affiliations of the new consultants, the presence or absence of established services in the private sector and the relative affluence of the local health authority. Generally, the new services have been able to set their own norms and establish innovative patterns of training and staffing. This paper documents what has been achieved in the southern half of one provincial Health Region. In addition, some of the guiding principles, problems and present solutions are presented.

Nottingham Then and Now, 1974 and 1989

The Nottingham NHS service was initiated in 1974 with my appointment. For 5 years I was the only appointed consultant medical psychotherapist in the Trent Region. Now there are companion units in Leicester (Chris Whyte 1979), Derby (Nassos Constantopoulis 1980–85, David Smith 1985) and Lincoln (Geoff Fisk 1985); a second consultant (Patricia Slack) was appointed in Nottingham in 1987. The Nottingham Psychotherapy Unit has nine full-time and five part-time members of staff drawn from all the mental health care professions and each working as a psychotherapist. It has the accolade of having a fully

From M.O. Aveline (1990) Developing a new NHS psychotherapy service and training scheme in the Provinces. *British Journal of Psychotherapy* 6, 312–323.

accredited senior registrarship in psychotherapy, provides a wide range of trainings and clinical services and contributes to the 3-year plus certificated South Trent Training in Dynamic Psychotherapy for career psychotherapists which is collaboratively provided by the four units. A consultant in behavioural psychotherapy (Alan King) was appointed in 1981 in Leicester.

In the beginning outside the NHS, there was little provision of psychotherapy, certainly of dynamic psychotherapy. Since the early 1960s, clinical theology had been developed in Nottingham under the charismatic leadership of Frank Lake, and in its practice was becoming increasingly preoccupied with hypothesised birth trauma, rebirthing and prebirth trauma. A transactional analysis centre was formed in 1976. A few general practitioners had Balint training and there was one experienced psychosexual therapist. To this day no analyst practises in Nottingham. The nearest psychoanalysts were to be found in Sheffield and Leicester and the nearest analytic psychologist in Lincoln. Among the citizens of Nottingham there was little familiarity with psychotherapy. Early on my patients used to refer to therapy sessions as 'classes', thus implying a passive instructor/instructed model which was alien to my purpose. Whilst there was little to draw upon in establishing my service, I had the priceless advantage, to my way of thinking, of there being no set pattern to constrain my efforts.

Non-NHS developments have been on three fronts: academic, institutional and private. London continues to be a magnet for training, though this is slightly offset by the introduction of centrally sponsored courses such as the introductory course of the Institute of Group Analysis which is held in nearby cities. Sheffield mounts a Diploma in Psychotherapy over 4 years part-time, and in 1979 the radical and highly successful MSc in Psychotherapy started at Warwick University. Universities and polytechnics have somewhat belatedly recognised their responsibility to provide assistance with the psychological problems as well as the academic ones of their students and staff, and have developed counselling services, most noticeably in Loughborough, Nottingham and Leicester. A parallel development has been of counselling services, open to self-referral and funded by local authority grants and means-dependent fees. There has been a veritable explosion in self-help groups and the culturally significant appearance of Women's Therapy Centres in Nottingham and Leicester. A small number of graduates of the new London private training institutes, skilled in the orthodoxies of analytically informed individual and group psychotherapy, have made their way to Nottingham. However, the growing band of private practitioners predominantly offers the more experiential therapies of gestalt, psychodrama and bio-energetics; local or nationally affiliated trainings in these approaches burgeon.

A Personal Note

Affiliations predicate the use that is made of the opportunities available to develop a service. Diversity in approach has characterised my training. I have been supervised in humanistic, Jungian, Freudian, object-relations and behavioural approaches. Outside the hospital, I was involved in the encounter movement and the creative therapies (Aveline, 1979; see Chapter 1). Latterly, I have been impressed by existential psychotherapy and the American interpersonal psychologies of Horney, Fromm-Reichmann and Sullivan. Indeed I now call myself an interpersonal psychotherapist; this means that, in my work, I emphasise exploring meaning and elucidating the narrative of interpersonal conflicts; I encourage the patient to accept responsibility for his actions and exercise choice. The breadth of my experience, together with the research evidence, has left me unconvinced that there is any one royal road in psychotherapy. There are a vast number of schools, similarly effective and seemingly different in approach, but having in common the same therapeutic factors (Frank, 1974; Aveline, 1984a). Though keenly aware of the comfort and security in being a member of a school, I have tried to pursue an integrationalist course. Integration does not imply assimilation for I recognise that therapists and patients have particular affinities for certain theories and approaches, be they deep or symptom-focused, and thus have sought to unite the right therapy and the right therapist with the right patient. One consequence of this approach has been the necessity to build a team whose members have different styles and approaches but who would respect each other.

For me, individual potential for fruitful living is limited by guiding fictions that a person has learnt or evolved to explain his or her actions. The therapist encourages the patient to take action that, once succeeded in, will rewrite the cramped fiction of his life. This good action challenges the view that has been taken of the person by significant others and by the person of him- or herself; it challenges the view which will be taken of similar events in life now and in the future unless some corrective experience occurs (Aveline, 1986; see Chapter 2). The encouragement the therapist offers may be covert, as in analytic therapy, or overt as in behavioural therapy. In the former, intrapsychic terrors are faced and the treatment proceeds by analogy; if a new end to the old sad story can be written in the relationship with the therapist, the same new chapter can be written in the natural relationships outside the consulting room. In the latter, direct action is taken, perhaps after a period of rehearsal, often undertaken with the therapist. The same direct action is a strength of marital and family therapies. What characterises good therapy is a sustained, affirmative stance on the part of an imaginative, seasoned therapist who respects and does not exploit (Schafer, 1983).

Patients with deep problems of self-doubt and negative world view need sustained care in order to change; it is this group, so common in NHS psychiatric practice, together with the NHS itself and, grandiose though it may sound, the nature of British psychiatry that have seized my energies. The original remit in Nottingham was to provide a tertiary clinical service to psychiatrists and to teach. I was happy with this, as for me psychotherapy is an essential presence within psychiatry.

The Early Days

Before I was appointed, one of the general psychiatrists in Nottingham had led a supervision seminar for a couple of years. In order to improve the standards among trainees, then of variable quality, the psychiatry training programme emphasised precise descriptive phenomenology and categorical diagnosis; organic treatments were much used.

I was intoxicated by the limitless opportunities to practise my skills and threw myself into organising supervision groups, shared clinical ventures, Balint groups and, possibly prematurely but not without value, participation in local and national committees. Within 2 years, I was the willing victim of my own enthusiasm and often felt like a juggler who has a number of plates spinning on the top of poles and needs to rush from one to the other to prevent any falling (Aveline, 1976). This pattern continued until quite recently.

To retain one's self-respect and the respect of one's colleagues, one needs to provide a sound clinical service, but clinical practice cannot dominate if one is to fulfil the intended major role of teacher of psychotherapy. As I have some talent for committee work, I determined to make a contribution outside psychotherapy in that sphere. Being on my own with offices in three sites, a half-time secretary and only two sessions from an experienced social worker imposed its own imperatives. I reminded myself that mighty oaks grow from small acorns and set out to do what I could. A supervision group became an advanced group after a year, and necessitated an introductory group. After 2 years, there were three supervision groups, a group therapy course, a Balint group, two out-patient therapy groups and a couples group, all of which required my presence. Very quickly I realised I needed supportive friends, both locally and at large.

Locally, I set up a support group of five experienced therapists. We met each month to discuss cases and consider training. Later, with colleagues from Leeds, Sheffield, Liverpool and Newcastle, we established the Northern Advisory Group which acted as a clinical and political support group to all therapists in the northern half of England. Seeing how each was tackling similar problems stimulated fresh thinking and encouraged us to keep going when progress seemed slow. My training and clinical innovations drew upon the services of the local group but were mainly supported by talented, fairly junior, colleagues of all disciplines, whom I invited to join me in some new venture. These were volunteers; they had the keenness of their enthusiasm but their presence was impermanent. They were like mini-teams, especially as I attached to each group therapy venture student observers or junior therapists in order to extend the training facilities. The common link was myself, which was arduous and meant there was no-one with a complete overview who could fully deputise for me in my absence. This and the growing number of difficult referrals whose therapy required experienced therapists engaged my energy in establishing staff posts in psychotherapy, initially shared with other services but later full-time.

Two practical points arise from this experience. Both relate to critical mass. In the first place, any successful organisation needs at its core a sufficient number of like-minded people who can support each other when the going is hard (as is often the case when the patients' problems seem unresolvable or the local professional climate is apathetic or downright hostile), who can generate and put into practice new ideas and who can confidently meet the clinical demands placed on the service. I suspect that the ideal number is around five, either in total or in subgroups; fewer and there is no space for individual dislikes to be dissipated without spilling over into warfare; more and the lines of communication become too long.

In the second place, in the long run, the core staff of psychotherapy units must be full-time and employed to work in the unit. In theory, two advantages stem from this: guaranteed availability and undivided loyalty. In planning, it is essential to know on whom one can rely. However, it must also be recognised that the staff alone will not be able to cope with the patient waiting list of a unit. Even if they could, this would be undesirable, as an opportunity would have been forfeited to draw others into psychotherapeutic work and so disseminate this vital skill into the wider arena of psychiatry and medical practice. It is necessary to involve trainees in meeting this demand. Initially in Nottingham trainees brought their own cases to supervision and, like most self-selected cases, they were horrendously difficult. Now all but a few trainees see Unit patients in the Unit, with the advantages of a lessened waiting list, better matching of patient and therapist, and the provision of a proper environment for the work.

In the early 1970s there were few senior registrars in psychotherapy outside London. I felt that a crucial element in developing NHS psychotherapy in the East Midlands was to have one in Nottingham. Two years of advocacy resulted in the first senior registrar, Mary Brown, taking up her post in 1978. Her successors have been Anne Goldingay, Jane Price,

Sue Gregory, Patricia Slack and Sophia Hartland. That early decision was undoubtedly correct. The central trainings have excellent features but their graduates are absorbed into career vacancies in or near the centre they rarely show a pioneering spirit and often imply that they would not wish to practise on what they see as the frontier without the refreshing company of others from the same regiment. Our graduates have a different outlook and their presence has given a major boost to developing our own specialist training scheme.

From early on, training has been multidisciplinary. To complement this, we needed multidisciplinary staffing and an appropriate building of our own to safeguard the practice of formal psychotherapy. The first was easier to implement; the second took years to achieve.

The Nottingham Psychotherapy Unit

The unit moved into a converted private house in 1981 and has now expanded into an adjoining building. The house is furnished domestically and provides a suitably informal and peaceful setting for the work. Within 10 minutes' walk of Mapperley Hospital (our parent psychiatric hospital), its location symbolises our separate identity *and* our willingness to be part of the whole.

Student and generalist training

More than half of each week is devoted to training colleagues in psychotherapy at one of three levels: students, qualified health care professionals with a generalist interest in the subject, and career psychotherapists. This is not the place to give an exhaustive account of the work of the unit, but for students a diet of lectures and demonstrations is provided. For several years, we mounted an experiential day for medical students (see Chapter 8) but this has lapsed through curriculum changes. At any one time, up to six final-year student nurses may take 1 year of one day per week elective track in dynamic and behavioural therapy; two student nurses may do 3 months full-time in behavioural work.

For those with a generalist interest, a sequence of training opportunities is offered. Beginning therapists in dynamic psychotherapy join the introductory psychotherapy year, a weekly seminar which provides in the first 6 months an introduction to theory through guided readings and to practice through role-plays. After evaluation by the year leaders, the trainees take on selected level 1 psychotherapy unit patients in individual therapy (level 2 is for therapists taking their second or third cases; the difficulty or political sensitivity of level 3 cases means that their treatment must be undertaken by unit members). In the second and subsequent years, trainees may join one of six multidisciplinary supervision seminars, each with four members. The supervision experience may be extended by joining the reading seminar and greater personal awareness gained through membership of the group course, the experiential group or personal therapy. At the end of each supervisory year, the supervisees and supervisors write structured evaluations of each other's psychotherapy work. Structured group reports and written evaluations are also used in the training of group therapists (see Chapter 14). After 2 years with one supervisor, trainees are encouraged to change groups in order to broaden their perspective or to strengthen some weakness in practice that the first supervisor has not been able to correct; supervisors are either members of staff or colleagues with training. Trainees seeing two or more patients may negotiate individual supervision. In addition, trained nurses, occupational therapists and psychiatrists may compete for elective single-discipline training placement in formal psychotherapy in the unit for 2, 3 or 5 days per week for 1 or 2 years.

Therapy is mostly of the once-a-week, face-to-face variety and is open-ended in duration, though cases seen by beginners will generally be for around 50 sessions. Sessions are tape-recorded for the purpose of supervision. A similar structure is being developed for behavioural and cognitive therapy.

Specialist training

At the career level, the shared ambition between the four units has been to develop an advanced NHS training in dynamic psychotherapy which could be available to staff of all disciplines, would draw upon NHS facilities and which would be taken without the trainee having to incur fees. The result is the South Trent Training in Dynamic Psychotherapy which takes a minimum of 3 years to complete. The central element is the practice of formal psychotherapy for a *minimum* of 8 hours each week, the work being discussed with a principal and at least two elective supervisors whose roles, respectively, are to provide continuity and depth throughout the training and to provide variety in perspective, mode and focus. The second element is concurrent personal therapy, which is available without payment from senior members of staff in other units who have been approved as therapists, or from independent therapists for fee; the third element is nine terms of academic seminars.

When trainees feel ready and have completed the eligibility criteria, they may ask to be examined by an assessment panel which makes a recommendation to the training committee on the award of the certificate. Clinical competence as a psychotherapist is at the centre of the assessment and is based on supervisors' reports, the candidate's casebook, a detailed written account of one or two psychotherapies with optional transcripts and audio- or video-recordings of two sessions, and an essay which reflects an area of personal enquiry or research in psychotherapy.

Clinical work is the dominant motif in the training; we expect our graduates to be competent practitioners of psychotherapy, someone to whom one could confidently refer a patient for treatment substantially without supervision. Like all evolving organisations, we have made mistakes and, certainly, we have tried to see the error of our ways. It is, perhaps, a sign of our growing confidence as trainers that we can begin to value our differences and not strive after a constraining conformity. This should better harness our energies and help trainees make a selective choice from among our strengths. The result, we hope, will be a fostering of individual talent and preference among the trainees.

A training such as ours, which is for NHS staff and which values the principle of necessary training being provided without fee, faces a tricky issue over NHS and private-sector personal therapy. The trade-off is between free therapy inside the NHS and the greater privacy of therapy in the private sector. The senior registrar can make a free choice as contractually the Region has to reimburse therapy fees in full. On occasions it has been possible to negotiate this on a personal basis for certain non-medical staff but, generally, paying fees is a significant though not an absolute obstacle to choosing a private therapist for staff whose salaries are low. Even if it were possible for all to pay fees, the choice is limited as respected private therapists working locally are thin on the ground; their numbers need to be increased. Staying within the NHS, whilst ideologically worthy, imposes its own constraints; the personal therapist is ruled out as a potential supervisor, the therapy may feel to be taking place too close to home and trainers are inhibited from having full conversations with colleagues who are acting as therapists for fear of compromising the therapy in some way. One way ahead is to develop swap arrangements with therapists in nearby centres outside the training scheme.

Outreach

Outreach is our way of facilitating the psychotherapeutic work of colleagues in the district. All the staff have time in their week to provide, on request, supervision, brief courses, co-work and leadership of staff groups. Ward and day-centre staff are the prime consumers of this service.

Clinical service

Psychotherapists are sometimes taunted that they are only interested in young, attractive, verbal, intelligent and successful patients

(YAVIS). Such luxury is relatively rare in NHS practice, where the walking wounded are the norm rather than the worried well. This bias makes it difficult to find sufficient straightforward patients for beginning therapists and dictates a reparative style of therapy of around 18 months' duration. Our major work is with longstanding recurrent relationship difficulties and severe intrapsychic conflicts. The dynamic side of the service receives 200 referrals a year, all addressed to the consultants; they are assessed by senior members of the unit, discussed in an assessment meeting and placed on waiting lists for individual (three levels of difficulty), group, couple, family or behavioural therapy; the 200 behavioural referrals that we received before recent financial cuts were assessed both in the unit and in sector teams.

In common with other psychotherapy units, we have not been able to solve the problem of excessive waiting lists. Three months to assessment and a further 6–9 months before entering therapy is too long. Solutions might be to limit the duration of therapy, be more selective or do more focal therapy; other more controversial options would be to increase our staff or institute waiting-list groups. Hitherto we have felt that, without totally disregarding our obligations to those on the list, we should do our best with those actually in therapy. This means that we have to explain to referrers and patients the tempo of our work and its rationale, though it must be said that acquaintance with the larger picture is meagre solace for individual need.

One innovation was the introduction some 7 years ago of questionnaires on biographical details and goals in psychotherapy which patients have to complete, however sketchily, before they are offered an appointment. The questionnaires served to introduce the patient to the perspective of psychotherapy by providing information about the nature of the personal work they were embarking on; the sequences of the questions was intended to arouse hope by looking forward from the present problems to how the person would like to be, to help identify areas of success and people in their life who might assist them in their chosen purpose, and to cultivate a reflective attitude by asking what fears inhibit them. A 1-year follow-up of a randomised investigation of the therapeutic value of these questionnaires (Aveline and Smith, 1986) has been completed and will be reported. For some, the questionnaires serve their purpose. Certainly they provide a helpful source of information for the assessor. As a screening test of motivation, they have reduced the no-show rate for the assessment interview from 25 per cent to 8 per cent without increasing the overall failure rate to follow through with the referral. We have, however, found that completing the questionnaires is burdensome for some and so have introduced a simpler form.

Multidisciplinary staffing

The unit is mainly staffed by full-time therapists of various theoretical persuasions. The dynamic work is managed by two full-time consultants, two adult psychotherapists (one formerly a psychologist and the other an occupational therapist), two specialist nurses, a social worker and sessions from a clinical assistant and a clinical psychologist. The behavioural section, which is an integral but recently developed part of the unit, was staffed by three specialist nurses but is now reduced through financial cuts to one with the other two fortunately finding specialist employment in sector teams. The Unit has a full-time specialist senior registrar in psychotherapy and offers a full-time 1-year placement for senior registrars in general psychiatry, which is accredited for training for consultant posts with special interest in psychotherapy. Last, but certainly not least, are one full-time and two part-time secretaries whose support is essential, and who, without formal training, carry a great deal of the actual work of the unit; they are in the front line.

All clinical staff of the unit have similar job descriptions; the one exception is social work, where the managers are so opposed to any hint of NHS hegemony that they have their own undisclosed contract for their member. The job descriptions define the work as psychotherapy and institutionalise the requirement to gain through the local arrangements the training necessary to discharge that role; clinical accountability is to the consultant who oversees use of time, psychotherapy standards and training. These contracts protect staff from redeployment or the eroding demands of outside superiors to undertake work that is not central to the Unit. They give formal expression to the intention that the primary identification of staff is as psychotherapists and as members of the Unit. This is not to sever links with the profession of origin, but to assert the principle of meritocracy of talent. Origins are not forgotten, as each team member is specifically charged with developing the psychotherapeutic skills of the profession whence they came.

Despite the unifying effect of common contracts, differences in power, money and status destabilise the system. While the Unit may prize the principle of meritocracy of talent, that reality is not fully reflected in meritocracy of reward. Staff pay for the same work varies widely, and is governed by the best grade that can be agreed with the powers that be in the hierarchy of that profession. Differentials between the professions result in the ludicrous situation where a staff member with senior training responsibilities may be paid less than those who are being trained. In a very interesting development, the Secretary of State at the DHSS has authorised the redesignation on a personal basis of a staff member in the Nottingham Unit as an adult psychotherapist; her background is in occupational therapy but her work in dynamic psycho-therapy could not be properly rewarded, absolutely or relatively to other Unit members, within the Whitley Council regulations. The current re-grading exercise for nurses has altered relativities and, unless further adjustments take place, may leave a legacy of bitterness.

Knowledge and research

Psychotherapy is a purposeful activity. Someone comes for help with recurrent relationship problems or core conflicts and can reasonably expect to be provided with the most facilitative and briefest therapy, given the resources available. Particularly at career psychotherapist level, I consider that a fully professional attitude includes a sympathe-tic, critical appraisal of what in theory and practice is dogma and redun-dant habit, and what is enduring truth. An ideal is to ask oneself again and again three questions: (1) What actually helped this patient? (2) Could the end have been achieved more expeditiously? (3) Was there anything done that was to the ultimate detriment of the patient?

While certitude is but one step on the path from the confusion of training to the healthy scepticism and skill of maturity, a firm base in a consistent set of theory and practice is a good beginning. This can then be tested by the stringencies of clinical practice, challenged by the insights of other approaches and illuminated by the depictions of life in novels, plays and poems. Another step forward is to learn from research, either from the literature or from conducting investigations. Modest studies in Nottingham have had a practical bent: a compara-tive trial of psychodrama and group therapy, the value of group therapy in the management of insulin-dependent diabetes (see Chap-ter 8), psychological intervention with RAF personnel who have sur-vived ejection (Aveline and Fowlie, 1987) and the therapeutic value of psychotherapy pre-assessment questionnaires (Aveline and Smith, 1986).

The consultant's role

It is a curious paradox that what first drew me to the practice of psy-chotherapy has become less possible as the Unit has grown in size. I suspect others feel the same when they groan about the number of meetings and the slowness with which the decisions are made. What attracted me to psychotherapy was the opportunity to work directly with my patient, relying on my own efforts and personality to assist the process of change. Now I largely work through others; I assist them in their work of assistance. Increasingly, my primary role is in creating a secure environment in which others will be able to do good work. This is an essential task which the consultant is well placed to undertake.

As the organisation has grown in size, so has the amount of time that has to be spent on maintaining the structure – keeping and upgrading posts, getting better facilities and administration. Without the infrastructure the service cannot flourish. Currently, we are negotiating for the Clinical Director to take on budgetary responsibility for the Unit with that rotating between the two consultants; this could give us greater control over our destiny. Building and keeping good relations with colleagues and managers is a vital part of the consultant's role. Their good opinion of the clinical and teaching service provided is one index of what one is trying to achieve, and helps the service grow. A unit needs good friends and good information. Above all in this medically led service, the consultant has overall responsibility for the quality of assessments, therapy and supervision in the Unit, authorises the taking-on of more senior roles by staff, and has a pastoral concern that they are not over-extended and have the training they need. Anxieties generated in the staff by the work or by the dynamics of the larger system of the institution have to be contained. Within personal limitations, the consultant endeavours to be a model of good practice, both inside the Unit and at large. As the seniority of the staff has grown, the original consultant functions of flag-carrier for and standard-keeper of the specialty are carried by team members who have delegated responsibility for areas of the work.

In Conclusion

NHS psychotherapy is alive and well in Nottingham and South Trent. Within a short period there has been a remarkable flowering of specialist psychotherapy. Now, with five consultant psychotherapists whose main interest is in dynamic or interpersonal psychotherapy, one consultant in behavioural psychotherapy and 30 non-medical psychotherapists, we have within a 25-mile radius in the southern half of the Trent Health Region the largest concentration outside London of professionals working wholly as psychotherapists. Each unit, as one would expect, teaches at student and generalist levels, but the concentration of resource makes possible the provision of specialist training in dynamic psychotherapy as part of the working week, within the NHS, and substantially without fee. This is a radical departure for the NHS, which for many years has relied on private institutes and universities for training.

Despite its tedious bureaucracy and its once more to be altered management structure, the NHS stands for an ideal which I am proud to serve and now find myself having to fight for: the ideal of equal access to appropriate treatment, free at the time of need. However imperfectly, the NHS provides the only feasible setting for the comprehensive practice of psychiatry. Apart from the constraint of the waiting list and our preference for weekly therapy, our patients can have the psychotherapy they need. Within psychiatry, specialist psychotherapy is an essential presence; it is the treatment of choice for some conditions and acts as the advocate of the psychotherapeutic attitude of mind that is fundamental to good psychiatric practice (Aveline, 1984b). I have tried to remain close to psychiatry, to provide a specialist clinical service to the more emotionally damaged patients who are referred to psychiatrists, and to teach necessary skills to all who work in psychiatry. This orientation has given a distinctive cast to the Nottingham Unit and is different from other colleagues, who see psychotherapy developing into an autonomous specialty, separate from psychiatry.

All services have their priorities. Ours is the NHS; top priority is given to referrals from psychiatry and the training needs of their staff, then general practice and general hospital specialties. After these come counselling services, social work and probation and, finally, private practitioners who seek training attachments. More senior local private practitioners affiliate to us for professional company and development. In Nottingham and nearby, the private sector is very much a minority force but has an essential role in providing personal and training therapy outside the NHS system. In this role there is much scope for development.

The Nottingham Unit, in common with the other units in South Trent, has developed multidisciplinary staffing which offers specialist positions in psychotherapy for members of all the core mental health care professions. This worthy aim is not without its problems. Some members of staff bring with them political and personal agendas which may be detrimental to the desired ethos; they may welcome the freedom to specialise but are suspicious of the medically led managerial structure and fear medical dominance. Open communication is a partial remedy but a more radical solution would be to institute 4-year training posts, which would allow colleagues to move on because they find that they are not suited to the work or they want a different structure, or simply wish to return to the mainstream of their profession of origin.

I look forward to the establishment of a new NHS profession of adult psychotherapy, open to all non-medical mental health care professionals with a career structure from training through basic, senior and principal to top grade. This would meet the need for appropriate identity, reward and status; it would emphasise the professional nature of being a psychotherapist. My only reservation concerns the weakening of ties with the different professions that make up psychiatry. It would be a great pity if the new profession of psychotherapy became elitist and saw itself as having little or nothing in common with those who are at the very least first cousins; this would only constrain the corporate vision of what it is to be a nurse, social worker, occupational therapist or other mental health worker. It would be unfortunate if one profession of origin was dominant in the new ranks and stifled the present limited opportunity for someone from another profession to develop specialist skills. It would be equally unfortunate if there was no-one on the staff of a psychotherapy unit who could speak the language of other professions sufficiently well to encourage them to develop their psychotherapy talents.

Should the new profession of adult psychotherapy be open to those without a basic qualification in one of the core health care professions? Talent as a psychotherapist is not the exclusive preserve of any one profession and a background in the humanities is a considerable advantage, but the prevalence of major mental illness and the complex interactions with physical illness and treatments necessitate, at the very least, familiarity with these problems. A modicum of familiarity can be gained from clinical attachments but this does not compare with a full training. For the time being, I favour reserving these posts for members of the core health care professions. I do not share Lawrence's (1989) enthusiasm for adult psychotherapy developing as an autonomous profession, as this path only leads to fragmentation and poor teamwork, especially in the NHS where the service is medically led.

Looking to the future, psychotherapeutic attitudes and skills need to be disseminated widely through psychiatry and medicine. One token of success will be a greater emphasis on psychotherapy in training and examination (Aveline, 1982). Such achievements will need to be fought for at every level. Then, maybe, the specialist psychotherapist will be able to revert to what I see as the proper role as expert therapist for difficulty problems, teacher and supporter of others engaged in the same kind of work at different levels and advancer of the specialty through critical reflection and research. Of the many challenges ahead, I single out two. We must try to develop the means to treat successfully those patients whose negativity of personality exceeds the limits of human benevolence as these patients are so destructive to themselves and others (see Chapter 5), and we need to develop a comprehensive model of how people change and then modify our practice so as to strengthen our interventions.

References

AVELINE, M.O. (1976). Organisation of psychotherapy teaching in an area without such a tradition. *Conference on Training, Association of University Teachers of Psychiatry*, Institute of Psychiatry.

AVELINE, M.O. (1979). Action techniques in psychotherapy. *British Journal of Hospital Medicine* 22, 78–84.

AVELINE, M.O. (1982). The MRCPsych examination: time for change? *Bulletin of the Royal College of Psychotherapy* 170–171.

AVELINE, M.O. (1984a). Books reconsidered: *Persuasion and Healing* by J.D. Frank. *British Journal of Psychiatry* **154**, 207–211.

AVELINE, M.O. (1984b). What price psychiatry without psychotherapy? *The Lancet* **2**, 856–859.

AVELINE, M.O. (1986). The corrective emotional experience, a fundamental unifying concept in psychotherapy. Paper presented at the Annual Conference of the Society for Psychotherapy Research, Wellesley College, Massachusetts, June 1986.

AVELINE, M.O. and FOWLIE, D.G. (1987). Surviving ejection from military aircraft: psychological reactions, modifying factors and interventions. *Stress Medicine* **3**, 15–20.

AVELINE, M.O. and SMITH, L. (1986). Psychotherapy pre-assessment questionnaires: form, content and therapeutic impact. Paper presented at the Annual Conference of the Society for Psychotherapy Research, Wellesley, Massachusetts, USA.

FRANK, J.D. (1974). *Persuasion and Healing*, 2nd edn. New York: Schocken Books.

LAWRENCE, J. (1989). Psychotherapy in the NHS: a new discipline and the need for a new professional structure. *Newsletter of the Association for Psychoanalytic Psychotherapy in the NHS* **5**, 4–6.

ROYAL COLLEGE OF PSYCHIATRISTS (1975). Staffing norms for a medical psychotherapy service for a population of 200,000. *News and Notes. Royal College of Psychiatrysts*. October, p. 4 and December, p. 18.

SCHAFER, R. (1983). *The Analytic Attitude*. London: Hogarth Press.

Chapter 16
The Nottingham Experiential Day in Psychotherapy:
A new approach to teaching psychotherapy to medical students*

The medical undergraduate curriculum tends to emphasise the technical aspects of medicine, but psychotherapy is one of the few disciplines taught that attends specifically to patterns of human relationship, reaction and feeling. It has a major contribution to make in demonstrating the importance of the human dimension in both illness and health. The contribution may be made on medical and surgical wards or, more commonly and as in Nottingham, during the psychiatry clerkship. How that contribution is made depends on the special nature of the subject, the time available, and the objectives set by the teachers.

Recent studies of factors influencing the choice of psychiatry as a career by medical students highlight an antipsychiatric bias among non-psychiatric members of the teaching staff, peers and house staff, together with a perception that the subject lacks scientific rigour. These negative influences are offset by directly seeing psychiatrists at work, and by having personal responsibility for patients during the clinical clerkship (Eagle and Marcos, 1980; Crowder and Hollender, 1981;

---

*Written with Jane Price.

From M.O. Aveline (1988) The Nottingham experiential day in psychotherapy: a new approach to teaching psychotherapy to medical students. *British Journal of Psychiatry* **148**, 670–675.

Nielsen and Eaton, 1981; Brook, 1983; Wilkinson, Greer and Toone, 1983). Psychotherapy may be deployed in both the elucidation and care of medical and surgical problems, but the recognition that it is an essential component in the training of psychiatrists, together with its usual placing within the psychiatry attachment, means that its successful teaching faces the same obstacles as psychiatry itself. The same solutions would be possible in psychotherapy, were it not for two features: the content of the work, its confidentiality, and the patient's sensitivity over the matters being disclosed, place a constraint on observational methods of teaching, whilst the timescale for change – 15 months – far exceeds the duration of the clerkship. Unless special arrangements can be made (see below), this precludes the student from taking responsibility for a patient in psychotherapy.

Communication skills can and should be taught (Sanson-Fisher and Maguire, 1980); once acquired, these persist (Poole and Sanson-Fisher, 1980). The American psychotherapist Bruch (1981) has drawn a parallel between the learning the patient has to do and that which the trainee psychotherapist has to do – both are engaged in an active process of reappraisal. The therapist comes 'to some living awareness of the significance and dynamic meaning of the interchange with the patient'. However, psychotherapy cannot be properly taught at second-hand; it requires a living experience to bring home to the student some of the subtleties, stresses and pleasures of working in this way with another person. Given sufficient time and resources, the training model pioneered at University College Hospital, London, and now implemented in the Department of Psychosomatic Medicine at Heidelberg University, is ideal (Sturgeon and Knauss, 1979; Garner, 1981). Students have the opportunity to take responsibility for a patient, and work with him for up to 18 months; the cases are selected by the Department of Psychiatry and supervised in groups of six. This supervised experience allows ample space to explore the distressing and tragic issues of living and dying, trying and failing, and sometimes succeeding, that are inherent in medical life. Given the 6 hours of curriculum time available in Nottingham, other innovative solutions were needed.

In this teaching, there are four objectives, each lending itself to different solutions (Aveline, 1984). The first is to acquaint the students with the nature and special perspective of psychotherapy. An appropriate way is some form of direct experience of the subject, either through supervised practice or through membership of a personal group, ideally over the entire duration of the undergraduate course. The second is to teach what psychotherapy is and what it can achieve, how change occurs, in what setting and over what length of time; here, case discussion and role-play are appropriate means. The third is to inculcate some knowledge of what problems to refer and when; this would be best achieved by a factual handout. Lastly, we need to facilitate basic skills of listening, 'being with' and counselling (Wolff, 1971); role-play and supervised practice are the obvious candidates for achieving this. The Nottingham experiential day goes some way towards meeting each of these objectives, but gives particular emphasis to the first and the last.

The Nottingham Day – Context and Content

Until the spring of 1981, medical students in Nottingham received four 1-hour lectures on psychotherapy during the 10 weeks of the psychiatry clerkship, in the penultimate year of training. In this classic format, information was undoubtedly acquired, but what was not conveyed was a practical understanding of exactly what happens in psychotherapy, or a sense of the pleasure and the responsibility that goes with working with another person, to help him or her improve the quality of his or her relationships.

The Psychotherapy Unit secured a whole day for psychotherapy, replacing the lecture slots. We now report our experience with 15 experiential days.

Our goals for the day are:

1. To acquaint students with our way of working in a personal way, so that they see the things we attempt to do and feel them, rather than simply hear from us about them.
2. To show what psychotherapy has to offer as a discipline, by increasing self-awareness and increasing sensitivity to the emotions present in any doctor–patient relationship.
3. To encourage students to see the value of spontaneity as a vital part of our work.

However, we do not see it as a form of therapy for students, and have no intentions of leaving people more disabled after the day.

By the end of the day, we hope that each student has an idea about the way our Unit runs, how we assess people as suitable for psychotherapy, how we decide on a particular form of psychotherapy suitable for that patient, and how we begin, maintain and end therapy. We aim to give them a taste of both individual and group settings, and to demonstrate in a practical way how the members of the unit work together.

We also aim to demonstrate to each of them that they have abilities to work in a similar manner with patients and to heighten their awareness of themselves as developing, unique people, within the common framework of being doctors-in-the-making. We seek to explore the dynamics of the group they already work in, as a practical demonstration of group dynamics. We aim to keep the group active and constructive throughout the day, moving from theme to theme within a definite timetable. We do not attempt to focus on any one individual for a prolonged period of time, although we do give a clear message to students that if any of them find our day disturbing, they can contact any member of the Unit afterwards to talk things through.

Four weeks beforehand, one of the team meets the students for an hour to prepare them and give factual information about psychotherapy and the day. Certain anxieties are allayed, though doubtless others are raised. Students are reminded that the day is a compulsory part of their training, and are asked to come in casual dress and with food to share for lunch. As part of our commitment to seeing things through, the requirement that each student should be present for the whole of the day is particularly stressed.

The content of each day is the product of the interests and concerns of that particular group of students on the one hand, and the preferred way of working of the staff members on the other. The day is adapted at is happens, to the needs of the students as they declare them and as we perceive them. Our boundaries are a start at 9.30 a.m. and a finish at 4.00 p.m., reserving time for the students to review and evaluate their day.

Typically, the day begins with interview skills enhancement, followed by an examination by the group of some common experience of medical student life; the latter generates more personal or intragroup themes, which are explored in the afternoon. In short, the day follows the natural progression in psychotherapy: as the staff are seen to be caring and respectful, so trust is developed; the events of the morning make possible the work of the afternoon.

Interview skills enhancement and basic concepts (1½ hours)

Numerous approaches have been tried. Video of an assessment interview or of components of the 'conversational model' of psychotherapy (Maguire et al., 1984; Hobson, 1985) have been viewed and discussed. Students have been asked to role-play breaking the news of death or terminal illness to relatives, or exploring the fears of a woman waiting for an operation for breast cancer the next day; the role-play may be videoed to facilitate detailed discussion. Alternatively, counselling exercises from Eagen's *The Skilled Helper* (1982a) have been used.

The students' attention has best been engaged when they role-play psychotherapy patient and therapist. A staff member chooses an incident from a current therapy, and coaches one student into the role of that patient and the other into being the therapist; the 'therapist' can ask for help from his peers if he gets stuck, or someone can substitute for him. Also, the action can be suspended to allow the 'patient' to give feedback of his feelings and reactions to the therapist.

Initially, the dynamics of the case are not made clear, as our intention is to provide an opportunity to practise listening carefully to another, being warm and empathic, and to discover that doctors are capable of at least unconsciously knowing what is going on in the relationship. This discovery enhances the students' self-esteem, and demystifies the subject. It is then possible to discuss the structure of therapy, the likely outcome, and through an examination of the fit or misfit between the feelings and reactions of patient and therapist, to introduce the concepts of conflict, transference and countertransference.

For this purpose, we have found it best to divide the group of 15–20 students into subgroups of 5 to 7. The work of the small groups is improved by having the student choose which staff members to work with and which colleagues to group with.

Common experience in medical life (1½ hours)

At this stage, we propose exercises that will draw the group together by sharing some common experience or task, but which also highlight how different people are in their aspirations and perceptions. Energy is mobilised by warm-up exercises, and then the focus is explored by exercises which tap the student's ability to think creatively and symbolically (Aveline, 1979; Brandes and Phillipes, 1979; Remocker and Storch, 1982).

A favourite exercise is the time warp. The members of the group picture themselves 1 year, 5 years and 10 years hence. Volunteer students demonstrate their perceived future through sculpting – relationships are portrayed by posture and distance. Often the goal was being a consultant, a literally exalted position, but debate would be provoked by others placing family or children to the fore. One female student reflected her delight in being useful and strong by accumulating such burdens of responsibility that she was forced to her knees at the 10-year mark; in vivid form, she was faced with vital decisions.

Graffiti sheets may be pinned up on the walls. At one end of the room, students can write up their expectations on day 1 of what medical school would be like; and at the other, their experience of how it has been. This leads on to dividing the students into two or three groups, each with a staff member as a resource person, with the task of devising in half an hour a dramatic representation of medical student life, which they then perform and discuss. Again, individual and collective experience is given conscious expression; the content of this expression is discussed in the section 'Being a Medical Student'.

A more task-orientated approach is to brainstorm emotional issues that the students have difficulty in coming to terms with. Debate produces a list of three items, which are then worked up into illustrative dramas in the afternoon. Issues from one workshop were: talking about dying, delivering an abnormal baby, feeling angry with and alienated from 'neurotics', feeling helpless in the face of enormous loss, being weak and powerless in the medical system but at the same time being expected to be in the front line, and having to get 'hard' and not liking it.

Personal, intragroup or task themes (1½ hours)

Depending on how the morning has gone and what mandate the group has given, more difficult areas can be explored in the afternoon; the least stressful approach is the task-orientated drama. Generally speaking, in order of increasing stressfulness, these are: secret fears, the magic shop, portraits, group-sculpting, sociogram and the persuasion game.

In secret fears, each member of the group (including the staff members) writes on a slip of paper a minor secret about themselves that they would be embarrassed to disclose. The papers are distributed at random. Sitting in a circle, each speaks of the secret fear as if it was his own; others may explore how the speaker feels about that fear. This is an exercise in empathy, not in detection!

In the magic shop, the customer may purchase some personal characteristic that he desires, by trading for it some characteristics that he already has. Much debate was sparked off by one female student who began by wanting to sell her ability to have children, but decided in the end that there was nothing on the shelves of sufficient value.

In portraits each student has half an hour to depict in paint the image he presents to the world; later, each explains the picture to the group. A variant is to have the picture discussed in pairs and then in the large group. The individuals and the group gain an insight into how a person sees himself; quite often, missing and valued aspects are pointed out by the group.

Group-sculpting is a flexible informative technique: students volunteer to sculpt the group as they see it. When one group insisted on sculpting themselves as an undivided mass, the staff drew on observations made during the day, and remodelled the sculpture to show a more separated group, with some connections stronger than others and some students holding more central positions.

In a sociogram, patterns of relationship within the group are indicated by answers to questions such as with whom would you go up a mountain, with whom could you argue, and who could you rely on. Answers are signalled by putting a hand on the shoulder of the chosen person or persons. The chooser and the chosen can be asked about the basis of the choice and about how it feels to be chosen.

These are powerful exercises which often make visible what was known and unspoken. While at the time some peripherally placed students have had their sense of alienation heightened, feedback some

weeks after the day has indicated that the group has been more aware
of their positions and has brought them in.

To be successful at the persuasion game requires a robust competitive nature. A circle of seated students are paired with a standing student behind each chair; one chair is empty, and the person standing
behind it has to persuade someone seated to come and sit on his or her
chair, while the standing person who might be left has to attempt to
dissuade him. The seated person is not allowed to speak until he or she
has made the decision to stay or go. Strong emotions are quickly stirred
– sublime happiness when you persuade someone to move, dark despair when the fourth person turns you down; personal styles, subgroups and relationships are highlighted, and students have the
opportunity to be merciful or punishing. This exercise requires sensitive handling, and it is often best for the staff to join in.

In the final half hour, there is an open discussion, when we aim to
put in perspective the experiences of the day. We discuss how and in
what settings the exercises are used, and answer factual questions
about psychotherapy. Sometimes the students feel too close to the day
to want to discuss the subject on a factual level; sometimes through
knowing of the approach at first hand, their questions are more search-
ing and well informed. We remind the students that they can contact us
for individual discussion of issues.

Being a Medical Student

We have now had the experience of working with approximately 250
students. The groups have varied greatly in ethos and personality, but
certain tensions in being a medical student have recurred.

Judging from the graffiti sheets, students come to medical school
looking forward to being useful, being intellectually stimulated, and
meeting a lot of people. Excitement and freedom – especially from
home and parents – are the keynotes. After 3½ years, many feel that
their individuality is not being encouraged and that they have to conform; they feel they have become boring. Consultants are stuck-up and
money is a prime objective. Reflecting what we suspect is a peculiarity
of Nottingham, a significant proportion have become fundamentalist
Christians, with that becoming their first priority.

In one most graphic visualisation, students represented the medical
course as a machine which wrenched their skulls open, scooped out
their brains, and stuffed in standard-issue ones. Representations of the
ideal course have emphasised greater choice, time to progress at different rates, time to take breath during the clinical period, and a personal relationship with their teachers. Some had achieved this, but a
disquietingly large proportion had not.

Despite our knowledge of teachers who embody a holistic approach to every patient, technology and hard facts seem to dominate the thinking of most students. Female students were more likely to voice and feel comfortable with the personal. Perhaps not surprisingly in view of their youth (the early 20s) they did not feel confident in handling emotional situations. Over 3½ years, some of their natural interest in people as people had been dissipated.

In the groups, being openly competitive was difficult, as this was seen as threatening to the cohesiveness of the group; yet many, if not most, of the students are intensely competitive and will belong to a profession which is, in itself, intensely competitive. Students were reluctant to open up divisions and areas of dissent, which is understandable, as they had to get on with their colleagues while the group was together; they have no choice in the composition of the groups to which they are randomly assigned every few months. Nevertheless, denial was a common way of dealing with conflict; though railed against by the students, conformity was very much part of their psychological make-up, and led them not to protest. Conversely, to declare that they had needs was problematic; they seemed to feel their own integrity as people was being threatened. Emotionally (and financially), most depended upon their parents, and seemed not to question this; perhaps it was another aspect of their conformism.

Evaluation

Three sources of evaluation have been tapped – immediate, end of clerkship and informal over the following months: the first two are more comprehensive. Whilst comment in open discussion is always solicited, systematic feedback is gathered by having the students complete an anonymous written assessment before they finish the day. At the end of the clerkship, all students complete a written evaluation, which mentions the psychotherapy day among other events.

The majority of the students find the day 'fun'; they enjoy the 'games' and feel loosened up by the activities, though a minority find the games absurd. However, they often do not see how the experiences they have had link with the intention of teaching them about psychotherapy: 'interesting, enjoyable, but not useful in furthering understanding (of psychotherapy)' was a typical comment. In contrast, a few recorded that it was the first time that they had talked in detail about the issues that face them as doctors; they learned that talking about problems helps to come to terms with them. Few felt engaged by watching a video; they were bored and alienated by what seemed unnecessary jargon. Role-plays, dramas, and group-sculpts caught their interest; they valued the opportunity to see the same situation from different people's points of view.

The students' overall reaction to the day took one of three forms. Some felt the day had gone just far enough and were satisfied with what they had seen and felt, some that it had gone more than far enough and had obviously been given food for thought, and some would actually have liked to take their learning about psychotherapy a step further. The use of the term 'fun' parallels these reactions: for some, it appeared to reflect a true feeling of relaxation and enjoyment, for others it was a defensive focusing on one aspect of the day to avoid considering its more personal and difficult aspects, and for yet others, it was a background experience that enabled important issues to be dealt with. Both staff and students considered that the day could be improved by holding a companion day or half-day soon after.

The day has already passed into the folklore of the medical school. New students have their perceptions of the day shaped by the old; this cannot be wholly bad, as very few boycott it. Graduates of the day remember the events, and indicate that the dynamics of their group have altered. Differences between students have been more openly acknowledged and worked with; closer links have been made with isolated students.

Discussion

The purpose of our experiential day is to give the students a memorable and enjoyable illustration of psychotherapy; we provide a reasonably safe space in which the students can attend to and explore aspects of their personal and collective experience. Our hope is that they will catch some of our excitement with this work, and our teaching is by doing rather than by describing; in this, we are moderately successful. As the psychotherapy team contains different disciplines and personalities, there was often animated discussion on how far to take the experiential element of the training day; this kept a fine 'edge' on the day, while allowing the exercise of reasonable restraint. Such a mixture in the team enhanced and enriched the day, and modelled a lively working relationship within a multidisciplinary team for the students.

Medical student training encourages the acquisition of facts, with a tendency to boil down each subject to a simple set of statements – what the subject is, how it works, the indications and contraindications for referrals. This is a legitimate need for practitioners, who will need to know in general about the resources they can tap for their patients; the required facts are embedded in the experiences of the day, for the student who can abstract them, but this is difficult for most. Whilst staff can see the significance of what is happening, many of the students perceive the events as meaningless happenings, rather than as illustrations of a special area of discourse. They lack the frame which would enable them to understand what is going on. Better preparation is needed: two instead of one pre-workshop seminar is one answer; a fact-sheet for study before the day is another.

The timing of the day in the clerkship is important. Preferably, it should be at the beginning of the psychiatry attachment, so that the work may be consolidated on the wards. We feel that one day is the minimum for this kind of experience, a second half-day or full day the following week would be advantageous. Ideally, the personal and patient care issues raised by the day should be followed up in small weekly discussion groups, led by psychotherapy unit staff or general psychiatrists. Much of the success is attributable to the extensive ex-perience the staff have of the techniques used and of working together; staff with different interests would need to evolve other formats.

We are aware that there is a narrow dividing line between what we are offering and therapy, but the students' fantasy is that they may be forced into the role of patients or labelled as having problems. This is neither our intention, nor our practice: students set their own limits for self-disclosure, and these limits are explicitly respected. Our assump-tion is that all people have choices to make in their lives and that studying the interactions between patients and doctors and within groups assists the development of professional competence. Our use of particular techniques with the students illustrates how we would use similar techniques in our clinical work.

Each group varies in its interest in matters psychological; within groups, there may be rivalries, or needs to defend certain self-images, which impede full use being made of the day. Giving the students the opportunity to choose their companions in the small groups and to determine the level at which their small group will operate facilitates the day. This has led us to experiment with having three separate tracks within the day, each led by a member of staff, which allows the stu-dents to be at their preferred level; however, it is much harder work for the staff, and precludes the students from seeing how we work as a team.

We are concerned that so many students have described their medi-cal course as stultifying and that their interest in people as people has been dissipated. We hope that this finding will be taken note of by course planners.

The nature of psychotherapy is slow work over many months to effect useful change in self-image and patterns of interaction. It could be argued that a single intense day gives a false impression of the subject, and might even encourage the instant answers to personal problems that psychotherapists so deprecate. For our part, we are satis-fied if the day raises questions in a way that stimulates the medical students to search for answers, and if they are once more appraised of the fact that the personal and the technical are indivisible parts of medicine. With some – probably those who are already open to the subject – we are successful; we need to investigate our failure to reach others; though systematic follow-up enquiries need to be made, we are not aware that any student has been harmed by the day. We regret the lack of opportunities to follow up our activities, and would prefer to provide a weekly forum for discussion over the 10 weeks of the clerkship and beyond, if possible. Meanwhile, the experiential day is an unusual solution to a common problem of limited curriculum time and insufficient teachers.

Acknowledgements

We thank Amanda Stafford and Myra Woolfson who have been co-leaders in the experiential day.

References

AVELINE, M. (1979). Action techniques in psychotherapy. *British Journal of Hospital Medicine* 2, 78–84.

AVELINE, M. (1984). Teaching dynamic psychotherapy to medical students: AUTP Conference 1983. *Association of University Teachers of Psychiatry Newsletter* Spring, 37–41.

BRANDES, D. and PHILLIPES, H. (1979). *Gamesters Hand Book*. London: Hutchinson.

BROOK, P. (1983). Who's for psychiatry? United Kingdom Medical Schools and career choice of psychiatry 1961–75. *British Journal of Psychiatry* 142, 361–365.

BRUNCH, H. (1981). Teaching and learning of psychotherapy. *Canadian Journal of Psychiatry* 26, 86–92.

CROWDER, M.K. and HOLLENDER, M.H. (1981). The medical student's choice of psychiatry as a career. A survey of one graduating class. *American Journal of Psychiatry* 138, 505–508.

EAGEN, G. (1982a). *The Skilled Helper*. Belmont, CA: Wadsworth.

EAGEN, G. (1982b). *Exercises in Helping Skills*. Belmont, CA: Wadsworth.

EAGLE, P.F. and MARCOS, L.R. (1980). Factors in medical students' choice of psychiatry. *American Journal of Psychiatry* 137, 423–427.

GARNER, P. (1981). Psychotherapy: experience as a medical student. *British Medical Journal* 282, 797–798.

HOBSON, R.F. (1985). *The Heart of Psychotherapy*. London: Tavistock.

MAGUIRE, G.P., GOLDBERG, D.P., HOBSON, R.F., MARGISON, F., MOSS, S. and O'DOWD, T. (1984). Evaluating the teaching of a method of psychotherapy. *British Journal of Psychiatry* 144, 575–580.

NIELSEN, A.C. and EATON, J.S. JR (1981). Medical students' attitudes about psychiatry: implications for psychiatric recruitment. *Archives of General Psychiatry* 38, 1144–1154.

POOLE, A.D. and SANSON-FISHER, R.W. (1980). Long-term effects of empathy training on the interview skills of medical students. *Patient Counseling and Health Education* 2, 125–127.

REMOCKER, A.J. and STORCH, E.T. (1982). *Actions Speak Louder than Words*. Edinburgh: Churchill Livingstone.

SANSON-FISHER, R.W. and MAGUIRE, P. (1980). Should skills in communicating with patients be taught in medical schools. *The Lancet* 2, 523–526.

STURGEON, D.A. and KNAUSS, W. (1979). The teaching of psychotherapy to medical students: an aspect of training in psychosomatic medicine. *Psychotherapy and Psychosomatics* 32, 212–217.

WILKINSON, D.G., GREER, S. and TOONE, B.K. (1983). Medical student's attitudes to psychiatry. *Psychological Medicine* 13, 185–192.

WOLFF, H. (1971). The therapeutic and development functions of psychotherapy. *British Journal of Medical Psychology* 44, 117–130.

Index